15 Minutes to Fitness: Dr. Ben's SMaRT Plan for Diet and Total Health

$4.00

"In my practice I treat many athletes and nonathletes, but common to both is that I try to find ways to help them through exercise. I also teach anatomy and physiology as well as exercise physiology at the college level so that future generations of professionals have a working knowledge, if not a passion, for exercise. I still use the SMaRT method of training to this day, and I have continuously trained for the last 40 years. I do it because it makes the most sense from an exercise physiology standpoint. I also continue to train this way because it works. That is the formula for a healthy lifestyle."

—Michael A. Minardo, D.C., M.S.,
Diplomat of the American Chiropractic Board of Sports Physicians,
Adjunct Assistant Professor Manhattan College,
Adjunct Assistant Professor College of Mount Saint Vincent

"I have known Dr. Ben since 1992 when he took over the clinic where I was working with a personal trainer for the two years prior. The system I was using was pretty much the same old program of three sets of ten of each exercise, three times a week. I thought my results were pretty good. Then Dr. Ben took over. WOW! What a transformation. With just two workouts per week at 20 minutes or less, I achieved far superior results. Now 22 years later, I still work with him twice a week to maintain what I have. "If what you are doing is working, keep doing it." Through years of research, he has referenced multiple scientific articles that substantiate the facts supporting his program. It is a welcome relief to see his approach to diet and exercise presented without the hype and gimmicks found in so many other programs. The SMaRT program is easy to understand, safe to implement, and sustainable to any age. It just works! Dr. Ben practices what he preaches as demonstrated by the degree of strength and tone he maintains to this day. Follow his logical approach to exercise with the commonsense guide to diet and you'll achieve the same. I plan on doing the same for the next 22 years."

—John W. Bass, MD

"Dr. Ben is one of the few true pioneers of the clinical application of resistance exercise to treat the chronic health problems that plague modern society. Whether its obesity, diabetes, arthritis, or the muscle loss that comes with aging, Dr. Ben has developed a sensible and rational approach to diet and exercise that works in concert with our physiology to produce remarkably dramatic and consistent results.

I first started working with Dr. Ben about five years ago as we (at Johns Hopkins University School of Medicine) sought to obtain National Institutes of Health funding to study the effects of resistance exercise on health, function, body composition, and quality of life among children with Juvenile Idiopathic Arthritis. His contributions related to the development of the exercise protocol have been essential to the ongoing success of our project. I have no doubt that if you would diligently apply the information contained in his book, you would systematically transform your health, physical capabilities, and quality of life. Read it, apply it and transform your body, health, and life!"

—Kevin Fontaine, PhD

Professor and Chair, Department of Health Behavior,
School of Public Health, University of Alabama at Birmingham, Adjunct Faculty,
Division of Rheumatology, Johns Hopkins University School of Medicine

"Dr. Ben is one of the rare exercise experts who truly is an expert. He is able to sift through and discard the endless nonsense in the field of fitness and offer his clients and students what is actually safe, true, and effective about exercise. His kindness and warmth for everyone, vast experience in the trenches, combined with his deep understanding of the field, makes Dr. Ben the guru's guru. From him I have learned so very much."

—Fredrick Hahn

Coauthor of *The Slow Burn Fitness Revolution*
Author of *Strong Kids, Healthy Kids*
and owner of Serious Strength Personal Training Studios

15 Minutes to
FITNESS

Dr. Ben's SMaRT Plan
for Diet and Total Health

Dr. Vincent "Ben" Bocchicchio

SelectBooks, Inc.
New York

Copyright © 2017 by Vincent Bocchicchio

This edition published by SelectBooks, Inc.
For information address SelectBooks, Inc., New York, New York.

First Edition

ISBN 978-1-59079-423-4

Library of Congress Cataloging-in-Publication Data

Names: Bocchicchio, Vincent, author.
Title: 15 minutes to fitness : Dr. Ben's smart plan for diet and total health
 / Dr. Vincent "Ben" Bocchicchio.
Other titles: Fifteen minutes to fitness
Description: First edition. | New York : SelectBooks, Inc. [2017] | Includes
 bibliographical references and index.
Identifiers: LCCN 2016031036 | ISBN 9781590794234 (paperback)
Subjects: LCSH: Exercise--Health aspects--Popular works. | Physical
 fitness--Popular works. | Weight loss--Popular works. | Diet--Popular
 works. | BISAC: HEALTH & FITNESS / Exercise.
Classification: LCC RA781 .B57 2017 | DDC 613.7--dc23 LC record available at
 https://lccn.loc.gov/2016031036

Book design by Janice Benight

Manufactured in the United States of America
10 9 8 7 6 5 4 3 2 1

To my family:

Marie (Mom), Bo (Dad), and my brother Les,
who would all get a kick out of my success and were
the basis for my curiosity and treating work as fun.
They are missed every day.

And to Cathy, Bert and Marian (Baldassano) Tracy, James,
Jay Jay, Mikey C., R. D., Speros, Cissy and Dickey, and
Ellie who were there for all stages of my life and career.
They are truly family to me.

CONTENTS

FOREWORD

I met Dr. Ben about 20 years ago when my wife told me about an exercise specialist that one of her doctors recommended. She said he was a real character but had an ingenious system of very effective exercise that took only 15 minutes, twice a week. She tried it and was hooked by the amazing results she got in such a short period of time.

Dr. Ben and I have discussed the problems of obesity and diabetes many times, and he has expressed his deep professional and personal interest in addressing these issues and has considerable expertise in these areas. We both share a special interest in kids when it comes to these concerns. We have done some work together to teach kids about these problems and plan to do more.

I know Dr. Ben has led studies called "SMaRT Kids," implementing his innovative SMaRT exercise and eating plan. His results, both in these studies and in his private clinic (Dr's. Fitness Center), have proven to be remarkable.

I have met and worked with hundreds of trainers and exercise people in my lifetime, but Dr. Ben stands out as one of the true experts in the field. He has worked with world class athletes and everyday folks of all ages with uncanny success for more than 40 years.

With regard to "walking the walk," I can tell you from many personal experiences that he can eat as much as any person I've ever met, and yet he stays lean and muscular as he approaches 70 years of age. He MUST be on to something!

This book is a culmination of a lifetime of practice and study, and the SMaRT system of exercise and diet that he explains can work to make anyone that uses it stronger, leaner, and healthier for a lifetime. I hope you will read this book and apply the valuable information in your lifestyles and that of your family and friends. It can really change lives.

—Charles Barkley
November 2016

INTRODUCTION

Do you ever feel like a hamster, spinning on a wheel in an endless loop and getting nowhere when it comes to your health and fitness? Are you working out regularly and cutting calories but seeing no real improvements? Does it feel like you will never lose those last 10 or 20 pounds? Or do you feel as if you simply don't have the time required to lose the fat and get into shape? Imagine if you could have the blueprint for the most efficient form of exercise to keep your body healthy and fit and an eating plan to satisfy hunger, taste, and health. Well, now you can. The best part? It will only require 15 minutes of exercise, twice a week, paired with a controlled-carb diet, and on the average, you will lose 10 pounds of fat within five weeks. It's hard to believe, I know, but it works—and if you read this book, I will not only show you how but also explain why. If this sounds like just another "new exercise secret," I can promise you it's most assuredly not. The foundation of my program is based on years of study, observation, and practice, and I have seen it deliver real, measurable results in the overwhelming majority of my clients.

I have spent the last 40 years in the fitness and health field, and as I approach 70, people are still shocked to hear that I only spend 14 minutes twice a week on working out. But it's true. With only 7 percent body fat, I'm often asked what my secret is and if I possess a "magic bullet." I guess my answer would be that my magic bullet is knowledge. And now in this book I will explain why genetically our bodies require simple and limited exercise exposure and how you can follow this optimal pattern yourself. The fact is that as humans we are hardwired to exercise our bodies in very specific ways to reap the highest level of health benefits. I will provide the simple scientific argument for why my combination of high intensity exercise and controlled carbohydrate eating is the most effective means for burning fat, so that you can better understand exactly why this works. Exercise and diet are the two most powerful tools available for attaining high levels of health and function, and I will show you just how little it actually takes to achieve a maximum response.

How I Became "The Guru of Fitness"

This book is really the story of my life from a young, highly touted athlete to a self-directed career that I've thoroughly enjoyed and for which I am grateful every day. I have worked with movie stars, supermodels, world record-holding athletes, Olympic Gold medal winners, major sports MVPs, royalty, and academic- and scientific-prize winners. But some of my favorite clients have been much less famous, such as the lady who wanted to get out of her wheelchair and did, the 84-year-old who wanted to play golf again and walk upright without pain and did, the woman who was always fat and became lean and happy, and the people who had the guts to try to stay young and vibrant and not succumb to the sentence of aging. I have personally worked with more than 10,000 people, but half a million people have benefitted from my program's application in one of many facilities.

I found a subject and career that has been entertaining and fascinating. I've lived the lifestyle that I describe herein and smile every day as a result. So this how I became The Fitness Guru, as many people in my field now refer to me. As a child, I was mesmerized with my father's set of hand-cast weights in my basement in Staten Island. He used them to train for the fireman's test in New York City, where he became a captain. After graduating from

St. John's with a pre-law degree, my dad was drafted in WWII and served two tours of combat duty in Okinawa. He wouldn't let me use the weights until I was 12, but I snuck a few lifts in when no one was looking. I've been fascinated ever since.

I was a good but only vaguely motivated student. I liked to play sports more than study, but I read everything I could get my hands on about exercise and physical training (still do). I surprised everyone, including myself, when I attained a number of advanced degrees in related fields, but no one was shocked when I chose this area for my profession. After receiving a degree in physical education from Ithaca College, I went on to obtain my masters degree in education, specializing in exercise, and then a PhD in exercise physiology and a second PhD in health services with a specialization in physical exercise. I also completed a postdoctoral program in body composition and weight management from Columbia University.

I've spent many, many hours thinking about the best way to address real, efficient, safe exercise (probably more time than a normal person should think about anything). I actually invented a system as a result of wanting to get the most out of my money. In 1974 after completing my master's degree, I opened the first independent Nautilus training facility in my hometown of Staten Island, New York and created slow resistance training. I had read everything I could get my hands on about Nautilus and had the opportunity to meet the inventor, Arthur Jones.

Since I was a 24-year-old just out of graduate school, living with my parents and driving my 1964 Red Volkswagen (popularly known as the "Hulkmobile"), I had the most important business decision of my life to consider. I had saved nearly $3,000 from teaching during graduate school, and I planned to open a training center. The dilemma: Use my money to buy conventional equipment (barbells, dumbbells, pulleys, and benches) or somehow obtain $13,000 and pursue my dream of opening the first real

Nautilus training center in the Northeast. My family generously loaned me the money, and I rented out some space in a converted factory building for $315 a month. My friends and family helped me paint and lay some carpet, and I found an old desk in the building. I was officially in business. My nautilus machines arrived, and I vowed that I was going to get my money's worth—everyone who entered my facility was going to train my way or not at all! By the time I was 27 years old, I had opened six training facilities.

In the middle of my professional career, I had three major projects under way: I owned and operated the largest fitness center in New York City, I was a principle and director of a cardiac rehab center, and I was a principle and exercise physiologist for an international back treatment center. In each case I realized that the majority of the patients, clients, and members had a common problem: They were too fat. That was when I decided to enroll in my second doctoral program, which focused on fat-related disorders and the role of exercise in that arena. So while I have real, hands-on experience training clients successfully, my academic credentials and knowledge of the science behind what works has had an important influence on my program.

How I Created Slow Training

Many people have asked me throughout the years how I created slow resistance training. What sparked the light that fueled slow resistance training? Make no mistake—there was no such thing as "slow" resistance training before I instituted the system in 1974. Well, believe it or not, it all began in a geriatric home. . . .

In the early 1970s Arthur Jones designed a revolutionary series of resistance machines called "Nautilus." They were, quite simply, a quantum leap from all that had been available prior to that time, and, as I mentioned, I found a way to invest in these machines for my own training facility. Arthur had designed a unique concept where the "cams" or pulleys looked like nautilus shells. They were not round but instead had an asymmetrical shape. Arthur proposed that this irregular SHAPE on each machine provided variable resistance, which perfectly matched the optimal strength curve of human anatomy. This was the "secret" to the most efficient exercise.

The initial Nautilus concept of training was to produce as much *power* as possible. That included maximum speed and training three times weekly with two or three sets per body part. I felt that the exercise was harder and more effective if I performed the movements more slowly, so I began to follow a more controlled, one or two sets per body part, weekly routine. I knew it was more intense—I could feel it in my body—and somehow sensed that it was the best way to proceed. I had all of my clients and patients train in a controlled, strict, no-nonsense manner, working each set to failure. I allowed only one set and only twice per week training. Everyone had to have a scheduled time to train and everyone made substantial progress. Then the light went on!

How was I going to get the best results and the most out of my machines? I thought that Arthur Jones, the inventor of Nautilus machines, had a great depth of knowledge about exercise mechanics and responses. He had no formal training but deep insight. All of us in the field were enamored with Arthur's ideas. I was very impressed with his writing. And he always wore long-sleeved shirts with the sleeves rolled up. I was in awe of everything about him. When I asked him how he developed the supposedly "perfect" Nautilus cams, he told me that he had visited a geriatric home and taken isometric measures of elderly folks performing different exercise movements. He reasoned that these results would represent "perfect," purely anatomical, natural strength curves. Simple, unadulterated human leverages would be represented, and from that he could create ideal cams or pulleys for his revolutionary Nautilus machines.

Then I had a brilliant idea (almost as brilliant as Arthur's shirt sleeves): If the Nautilus cams were designed based on isometric (zero speed) strength calibrations, then the *only* way to take full advantage of my $13,000.00 investment (all I had and could borrow) would be to exercise at the speed that came closest to zero! Isometrics involve *no* speed. Also, the differential between the positive (lifting) and negative (lowering) phase of the exercise would be close to zero (in theory) during a close to zero speed or *very slow* repetition. In practice, at a minimal speed my machines would be best utilized. That was my thought process—the "germ" that generated my creation of the SMaRT system and ALL slow training.

Why I Wrote This Book

I decided to write a book because I see so many people struggling with their health, weight, and appearance, and there is so much misinformation out there. Many sincerely try to do the "right thing" and get nowhere but discouraged. I'd hoped someone would provide relevant, practical information about diet and exercise in one book but, in my opinion, it hasn't happened to my satisfaction. So, instead of spending more time on my golf game, I've put together some observations after 40 years of clinical practice and some sound, applicable science presented in a simple manner. Too many people don't realize that with the right program they can spend only 15 minutes twice a week to get their body back into the best shape possible.

If the national objective of promoting a lifestyle of diet and exercise has been the reduction or management of health issues—including obesity, overweight, diabetes, and a number of related problems—then even the most delusional of observers must conclude that the last 40 years of our history has been an abject failure. The numbers have spoken volumes for themselves:

- 78.6 million US adults are obese.

- As a result of obesity, heart disease, stroke, type 2 diabetes, and some cancers are the leading causes of American death!

- Over the past 35 years, the rates of obesity have *doubled.*

- The additional health-care costs for obese people annually are in excess of $1,400 per person!

- Pediatric type 2 diabetes has increased more than 33 percent in the past ten years.

These are epidemics directly related to overweight and obesity.

Clearly the diets and exercise commonly prescribed can't, by description, "work," or we would all be much healthier and in better shape. Many folks give up on diets and cease trying because they encounter a repeated, personal history of failure. While diet and exercise can certainly have a powerful impact on our health, it has to be the *right* kind of diet and exercise. It's like using "liquid" to put out a fire. Water may extinguish the flames, but gasoline (another "liquid") would have the opposite effect. In the same vein, the types of diet and exercise commonly applied to combat our health and functional problems are, in my mind, analogous to the gasoline choice for fire prevention. The purpose of this book is to simply describe the rationale for the most efficient combination of diet and exercise specifically designed to address these pervasive health problems.

In mid-2013, the AMA designated obesity as a disease. To some of us, this was *not* earth- shattering news! Why is this problem so widespread and what is the solution? Everyone knows that all you have to do to lose weight is to eat less and exercise more, right?

WRONG!

Perhaps no other issue is so misunderstood by the public and misrepresented by the scientific and medical communities, the government, and all sorts of "experts" who purport to "know" what's really going on. Americans are great consumers and willing to believe what they want to, often buying into the latest, greatest, easiest, most guaranteed plan to lose weight and get "buffed" with no "dieting" and some form of "magical" exercise routine. "Try this special berry extract," or listen to the TV doctor who has advice about a new twist or "discovery" every other week. Complete this enormously demanding exercise regimen to achieve a "hard body" like about one out of every 1,000 who live through the rigors of the unrealistic ritual do. These are the survivors you see on the infomercials. Who, in their right mind, can actually believe the claims reinforced by photos of these exceptional specimens will apply to them?

So why are we inundated with so many programs and plans and systems of exercise? And why is there a "new" and "revolutionary" system introduced every three months?

BECAUSE THEY DON'T WORK!

New crap replaces old crap. Many of these plans are simply unrealistic and impractical. Most are just plain ridiculous and ineffective. So, buyer beware when it comes to diet and exercise plans. History is laden with hundreds of scams and claims in these fields. If it sounds too good to be true, it probably is. However, if any system or program can identify some simple, reasonable science as a basis of its foundation, it might have some value or at least lead you to be willing to investigate its merits.

Where do we find legitimate information? The intention of this book is to provide an unbiased, simple, scientific source for objective answers. How do we begin to correct this unsustainable cascade of metabolic—or fat-related—problems and disorders? At the current rate, our kids will have shorter life spans than we will. Our health funds will run out of money while we become fatter, sicker, and less productive. This is not a radical version of the circumstances or the expression of some fear tactics; this is simply the trajectory of our last 40-plus years of behavior. We are more than 25 pounds (per person) heavier than we were 40 years ago. We are experiencing an epidemic of obese six-month-olds! This can't be acceptable. We must learn a better way to take care of our bodies and our health, based on sound scientific research and a program that has proven results for more than 40 years. It's not too late to take back your health.

A SMaRTer System

I wrote this for people who want to have a basic understanding of the principles that constitute a smart, healthy diet and practical, productive exercise plan. My program is the natural progression of a lifetime of study and clinical practice that started with the simple objective of finding "perfect" exercise. While it began with the development of a revolutionary program designed for elite athletes, it has morphed into a system of health and well-being applicable for anyone at any age or fitness level. Here are some of the logical components that I believe must be present for a highly beneficial exercise regimen and that are all present within the SMaRT system:

- **Safety:** Can it be done without injury, damaging inflammation, constant fatigue, or discomfort?

- **Simplicity:** Can almost everyone understand the basic principles involved?

- **Efficiency:** Can it be completed in a time frame that can be readily adapted into most modern lifestyles?

- **Universality:** Can it be performed by most folks at any level?

- **Effectiveness:** Does it accomplish that which most people want?

Everyone knows that exercise is good for them, but many people don't have the time or ambition to do it. Many others give up on repeated attempts at exercising, because they don't see results. Unfortunately, there are too many complicated, difficult programs out there that simply don't work for most people. There are thousands of "exercise plans" that claim they will give you the results you're looking for with little time or effort, but the majority of these fail at accomplishing real benefits. This leads to discouragement, which often leads to quitting. The three most common reasons (excuses) for not exercising are:

1. "I don't have the time."

2. "I'm afraid I'll get hurt."

3. "I don't see any results."

This book presents an enormously successful exercise plan that:

1. Takes 15 minutes, TWICE a week.

2. Has NEVER caused an injury in more than 40 years and tens of thousands of workouts.

3. Produces results in less than one month (performing eight 15-minute workout sessions in a month).

In 1974, when I created my slow resistance training program now called SMaRT-Ex®, it was originally designed for elite athletes whose time and energy were at a premium, especially during their competitive seasons. It has now been used by half a million people. So what exactly is "SMaRT-Ex"? Well, it's an acronym for **S**low, **MA**ximum, Response **T**raining **Ex**ercise, and it's a system I invented and developed that is now a mainstream fitness technique used by trainers worldwide. One of the most effective, efficient forms of exercise ever invented, SMaRT-Ex includes the following features:

- **S**low – Usually 15 degrees per second or slower (a much slower speed of movement than normal). This controlled speed allows for isolation and focused muscle loading (significantly slower than the common speed of resistance training).

- **MA**ximum – Unless a subjectively high level of demand is met, optimal exercise stimulation is impossible.

- **R**esponse – Constantly loading a muscle through its range of motion, using appropriate resistance to induce fatigue ("muscle failure") for a physiologically determined length of time, consistently produces the desired metabolic responses.

- **T**raining – Consistency and organization are mandatory in order to separate random physical activity from formal exercise.

My current program instituted decades ago is based on a circuit of resistance exercises performed twice a week with at least two days rest in between sessions. The large muscles are worked first, progressing to smaller muscle groups. For example: hips, legs, torso (lats), shoulders, chest, arms. It includes approximately six to ten exercises, and all movements are performed slowly and continuously, with the muscle groups generally under "load" for 45–120 seconds. When muscle failure is reached—the inability to perform another repetition in good form—the set is completed. Part II will cover my five-week metabolic makeover in detail.

There is real science behind why short, high intensity exercise works so well, and I will explain it to you so that you understand how your body is programmed to respond to it. I will also reveal why certain foods lead our bodies to burn more fat and how following a controlled-carb diet will maximize your success by giving your body exactly what it needs. The intensity, duration, and frequency of exercises in what I now call my SMaRT workout program have been designed to achieve optimal results not only for muscle strength and fat loss, but also for improvement in overall health and well-being.

My former client Gary is a great example of exactly how this program works. He was a 66-year-old who had been an elite level, masters group distance runner. An avid runner—and a longtime vegetarian—he had remained lean and in great shape for years. When Gary suffered a hip injury, he had to back off from running. As a result of that and some laxity in his eating, he found himself heavier than at any time in his life, weighing in at 170 pounds. Gary began doing his Total Gym SMaRT workouts and decided to restrict carbohydrates in a serious manner. He did this on his own, at home, keeping records of his exercise/activities and eating numbers (carbs, proteins, and so on). He cut his carbohydrate intake to fewer than twenty grams per day. Adhering to the SMaRT twice-a-week exercise program and the SMaRT low-carb eating plan, Gary transformed from 170 pounds to 155 pounds in 10 weeks and dropped two pants sizes. This got him back into trim running condition and improved all of his lab numbers in his annual physical at age 66.

• • •

The fields of diet and exercise have been historically rife with contrived methodology, bad science, and bizarre applications sold to a desperate public. It might be comical if it weren't for the millions of people who wasted hours and dollars on bad plans promoted by folks who should know better (government, powerful corporate industries, and lazy—if not negligent—scientists).

No one at any level or age wants to waste any time or effort on an exercise program. When I designed the SMaRT system, I wanted to cut out all the wasted effort and maneuvers in exercise and only include those elements that actually produced some positive response or benefit. Embodied in the SMaRT plan is the goal to only perform exercises that produce the highest return with minimum risk or damage.

After many years and many calls for this book, I have decided to provide the overwhelming evidence that the so-called "healthy" advice we've been given has been the very cause of our declining health and wellness over the last 40 years. Not without fault are the "experts" who denigrate either diet or exercise, while riding the notion that one without the other is really the answer. The SMaRT system is a synergistic plan that combines exercise and diet in a powerful combination in order to produce the biggest bang for the user's buck.

As a word of advice for the reader: If you follow the recommendations contained herein, you might become threatening to your doctor, family, and sincere friends who think they have your best interests at heart. The alternative "plan" hasn't worked and the time has been long overdue for dealing with good science and the reality of basic human physiology.

No one, including me, has created new pathways, chemistry, physiology, or anatomy, but enough bona fide information is available upon which a sound, simple, and practical behavioral plan can be structured. Never accept any advice dealing with your health and well-being without doing your homework. Be your own doctor, dietician, and trainer—or at least become an informed consumer of these disciplines. This is not only a personal choice but also a national necessity for a productive, healthy future for all of us and our children. Treat these decisions as if your life depends upon them . . . because it does.

PART I

Why Exercising and Eating the SMaRT Way Works: Our Physical Foundation

CHAPTER ONE

MUSCLES CAN'T COUNT: EVOLUTION AND SCIENCE

To better understand why the SMaRT program works, we need to travel back about 2.5 million years. Yes, it's true, I've been around a long time, but even I have to rely on what anthropologists have reported. Physiological and anatomical anthropology reveal that the current physical state of the modern human species evolved over a period of more than two million years. It seems that the human body and its chemistry are based on behaviors that allowed our species to succeed by developing certain "survival" characteristics. Those who didn't adopt these behaviors became, well, extinct.

To be more specific, if you think living in prehistoric times was not physiologically and metabolically challenging and was an easy deal in any way, please reconsider. It was enormously dangerous and demanding. Try living on your own for a week without *any* help or tools for getting food, water, and shelter—and getting away from many animals that have access to eating you and your family! It's drastically physical ("life or death" type) and demanding. Food can be scarce or at least only available sporadically.

As a result, we had to develop physiological "systems" to generate and support our search for and capturing of food and avoiding our predators. These systems included cardiovascular (heart and blood vessels), respiratory (breathing), endocrine (hormone), skeletal (bones), and nervous (brain, spinal cord, nerves). They all developed significantly to support the needs of the *Muscle System* and resulted from the demands that drove our health and evolution.

Why Our Bodies *Need* Exercise

So what does this all mean for our current health and well-being? It means simply that the human body *requires* significant physical stimulation (activity/exercise) in order to attain and maintain natural levels of optimal health and functional capacity because of how our bodies evolved millions of years ago. Since we no longer have to hunt and chase, run for our lives, and do without food for prolonged periods, our daily lives are obviously different than they were in the first two million plus years of our development.

However, even though our lifestyles have been altered dramatically, and many of us work in offices instead of hunting outside, the evolution of our physical bodies has not caught up to our modern-day habits, and therefore we are still wired to be most healthy when we are engaging our muscles in a high intensity way. The body operates by sending signals to and from cells, tissues, and organs. So we have to learn to adopt the behaviors that fit into our modern lifestyle that will still send the signals that drive us towards health and negate the signals that drive us away from that state of well-being.

How do we do this successfully? Here's my take: First, it has to be safe (no need to cause harm when trying to promote benefit). Second, it has to be universally applicable (good for just about everyone). Third, it has to work quickly and consistently (we are a very impatient species). Fourth, it has to fit into a modern lifestyle. And fifth, it has to provide as many benefits as feasible in one simple package. Is that magic? No. It's a basic plan that makes sense and has worked for tens of thousands of people in every type of population (be it old or young, men or women, fit or sedentary).

It is true that we can't do much to change our genetics, but we can affect our environment through our selected behaviors. Among the two most powerful human behavioral "signalers" are appropriate exercise and diet. So what is the best exercise and diet program to give us a shot at high health? It's the SMaRT plan. It's not about hours of cardiovascular exercise like running or multiple repetitions on numerous machines. It's about working your muscles in an optimal way that will ignite the body's signals for health. It's also not about counting calories but about eating the foods that will work best with your body's chemistry (more on that later).

Muscles Can't Count
(But They *Can* Send Healthy Signals)

I can't count how many times I have told people that *muscles* can't count. I say that because the number of sets and repetitions isn't that important. In reality, muscles only know how hard you're taxing them (intensity) and for what period of time (duration). The rest is really on automatic pilot. The support systems now take over and try to meet the demand that the exercising muscles are dictating. If we send the right signals through our exercise movements, the body, in a reasonably healthy state, will respond positively. Easy, right? Not so fast grasshopper!

Just what are these "good" signals? In overly simplified terms, these are the pathways that instigate just enough upheaval to coerce the intended systems to adapt upwardly and not enough to cause other unintended problems that are nonproductive or even counterproductive. There is a small window between stimulating positive muscle response and simply working at a level that might cause fatigue and sweating but doesn't drive a substantial change in body chemistry. Therein lies the magic (to many, it must seem like that).

Remember that we humans had to exert great amounts and bursts of energy to seek, capture, and finally eat our food (our energy source). We had to run, jump, climb, and hide from predators and seek refuge from the elements. Those are simply the facts of early human survival. That scenario involved the necessary capacity to produce enormous muscular effort and support systems to allow that muscle work to occur.

In almost every case, the benefit derived from exercise relates to the focus and intensity of the muscular effort. That, in turn, has everything to do with the types of muscle fibers that are stimulated to their respective threshold levels—when they start to actually turn on the body's signaling (we'll discuss more about muscle fibers in chapter three). In simple terms, the energy pathways, types of muscle fibers activated, and the corresponding responses can be expertly manipulated for our benefit. I will illustrate why relatively little exercise is required to derive maximal benefit and that *no amount of low level exercise or activity can substitute for that specific, high intensity muscle recruitment pattern*. With regard to productivity of exercise, LESS is almost always MORE! I think that's GREAT NEWS for everyone. Productive resistance training turns on the right signals to drive the most beneficial responses from our bodies so that they will burn calories and fat. When it comes to burning and storing fat, what we choose to eat is equally important for producing the signals that are associated with positive responses and results.

Storing Sugar for Fuel

Glycogen is a singularly important element to consider when thinking about how our bodies operate effectively. It's the form of carbohydrate or package within which the body stores glucose or sugars—mainly in the muscles and liver—available for quick fuel responses. The body can only store a limited amount of glycogen healthily, and the rest circulates in the bloodstream or must be converted into fat for safer storage (not a great necessity unless famine occurs). However, since glycogen fuels our "fight or flight, life or death" muscle fibers, our body considers its absence a serious situation (serious because if it is depleted, we have no "backup" to fuel potentially life-saving actions). Even the perception of depleted glycogen triggers emergency adaptations. We can control glycogen signaling with controlled-carb eating and high intensity exercise. Controlled carbohydrate eating enables our bodies to maintain essential glycogen stores in the muscles and liver (where it healthily belongs) by converting the body to a primarily fat-burning machine. Lowering carbs also reduces the levels of insulin necessary to drive sugar into muscle cells.

The healthy storage sites for glycogen are the skeletal muscles and the liver, but these organs have a limited storage capacity. When more carbohydrates (sugars) have been taken in than can be handled by the muscles and liver, the body has no choice but to drive them into storage in the form of FAT. This is even more evidence that the regulation and control of glycogen storage and usage is a vital mechanism when we are trying to lose fat.

We use our "fight or flight" muscle fibers when our brains sense emergencies or physically special events. We also draw upon our "highest octane" fuel—glycogen—so that we can drive the highest level of muscle contraction. Our bodies remember these events and try to compensate by increasing muscle and energy potentials for the next emergency. When we engage in high intensity exercise, it signals a depletion of glycogen, and the healthy response is for our bodies to attempt to replenish it at a higher level for the demand the next incident might require. As a result, we should be able to generate more strength and store more glycogen in our muscles (versus turning it into fat) in the best, simplest future scenario.

How does the everyday Joe or Jane accomplish this type of high-level chemistry and its many associated benefits? The simple answer is high intensity muscle stimulation—or high intensity slow resistance training. That may sound ominous and unachievable for many regular folks but, in fact, it is not at all! Remember, the "high intensity" aspect of exercise is subjective. It means that what might very well be high intensity for someone who has been sedentary will not be for the elite athlete. However, each is striving for the same relative level, requiring the body to respond and adapt "upward." You may start with very little weight or resistance, but it will gradually increase throughout your program as your body adjusts and gains strength.

Hormones and Weight Control

There are a few significant chemical pathways related to weight control and fat metabolism. If we can influence insulin, glucagon, and leptin through our behaviors, we have a much better shot at controlling our metabolisms. Insulin is a hormone we want very much to control, because it is the direct response hormone (chemical molecule) to eating carbohydrates. Insulin drives fat storage and inhibits fat release (burning).

We discussed how the body sends signals back and forth, in cycles, to regulate, initiate, and inhibit all sorts of physiological actions and reactions. The balance or net effect of all these activities ideally constitutes a condition called homeostasis or equilibrium. In the case of energy regulation—whether we are burning fat or storing fat—two of the most important signalers are insulin and glucagon. When the body produces too much insulin, it causes myriad problems, including obesity, high blood pressure, inflamed arteries, metabolic syndrome, and full blown type 2 diabetes. In its wisdom, the body does have a counterbalance to insulin in the form of a hormone called glucagon. When these two are functioning in an appropriately healthy coordination, usually all is well with our health status. A healthy balance between these two hormones is vital for optimal health and energy control.

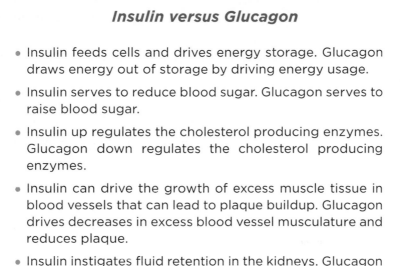

Insulin versus Glucagon

- Insulin feeds cells and drives energy storage. Glucagon draws energy out of storage by driving energy usage.

- Insulin serves to reduce blood sugar. Glucagon serves to raise blood sugar.

- Insulin up regulates the cholesterol producing enzymes. Glucagon down regulates the cholesterol producing enzymes.

- Insulin can drive the growth of excess muscle tissue in blood vessels that can lead to plaque buildup. Glucagon drives decreases in excess blood vessel musculature and reduces plaque.

- Insulin instigates fluid retention in the kidneys. Glucagon draws fluid out of kidneys.

- Insulin drives sugar energy use. Glucagon drives fat energy use.

Insulin Sensitivity and Resistance

Most of the problems associated with higher carbohydrate intake are insulin-related. Insulin is the hormone that regulates the amount of sugar in the blood. Our bloodstream only carries about a teaspoon's volume of sugar in the bloodstream at any given time. That very specific amount of blood sugar MUST be controlled within precise limits. If blood sugar gets too high (through a lack of insulin production or the inability to use the insulin present), we can get nauseas, short of breath, and in extreme cases, it can cause death from something called ketoacidosis. If blood sugar is not regulated through insulin and it falls too low (hypoglycemia), it regularly causes blurry vision, rapid heart beat, morbid fatigue, trouble thinking clearly, and unconsciousness.

Insulin sensitivity simply refers to the level of response that the insulin receptors (mainly in the muscle cells) have to using a normal concentration of insulin to do their job of absorbing energy and nutrients. Insulin resistance is simply the inability of the cells to respond healthily and appropriately to insulin exposure. If the cells become insulin resistant, they require more and more of this powerful hormone to accomplish the job. Problems arise when carbohydrates instigate a continuous drive for insulin production (secretion).

When this condition continues, the muscle's insulin receptor sites simply become insensitive or resistant to insulin's presence. What this means is that energy cannot enter the cells readily and the cells must either be exposed to increased insulin levels or the energy must be stored somewhere else. Usually, that somewhere else proves to be an unhealthy accumulation in some organs or tissues that become overwhelmed by the excess. Therefore, insulin sensitivity is at the opposite end of the spectrum from insulin resistance. Healthy insulin sensitivity refers to a quick and efficient response to insulin by the proper storage of sugar (energy). Insulin resistance refers to a muted or blocked level of healthy energy storage driven by insulin.

Even the most shortsighted nonbelievers regarding the value of exercise related to fat loss have to agree that exercise increases insulin sensitivity (a very good thing). By controlling the insulin response to carbohydrate eating, the regulation of fat usage and storage can be directed toward the fat-burning mode rather than the problematic fat-accumulating status.

The two most powerful mechanisms for controlling insulin-related problems are low carbohydrate eating and muscle building exercise. How does this work? By eating fewer carbohydrates (especially sugars and refined carbs, such as white bread), the amount of insulin secreted is reduced, allowing for a more preferential "burning" of fat for fueling. Remember, the sugars contained in carbohydrates (sucrose, fructose, and so on) are stored in bunches called glycogen, and that the healthy storage level of glycogen is limited.

In addition, carbohydrate or sugar "cravings" are consistently reduced when blood sugar is kept at lower levels by minimizing the fluctuation of the carbohydrate/insulin axis. High intensity exercise actually demands that muscle glycogen is tapped and readied for the "emergency" scenario that that level of muscle action/demand dictates. This triggers the release of stored fat for potential energy backup. As a result, the insulin receptors at the site of the working muscles become more responsive to regaining their glycogen status for the next "emergency."

The healthy body always tries to compensate for deficits encountered. So if the muscles are too weak for the demand imposed upon them, they compensate by getting stronger. If the bones are stressed positively, they grow denser. If the insulin receptors at the site of the working muscles are "threatened" by depletion, they compensate by taking in fuel (blood sugar) at a higher rate to reduce the possibility of being in a deficit situation the next time it might occur.

The Facts About Insulin

- It blocks leptin in the brain, so you feel hungry all the time.
- It drives fat into storage, even when you are tired and need it for energy.
- It trumps other hormones, except for glucagon.
- It makes you more carb "sensitive."
- It is absolutely driven by carb intake.

Leptin

Regardless of the method or philosophy applied to diet, we must consider hunger or the drive to want to eat. Satiety, or the sense and feeling of fullness, is the counterpart to hunger. Interestingly, these sensations are significantly controlled by a hormone called leptin.

The real importance of leptin lies in its deficiency, which is associated with obesity or weight gain. In obese rats, when leptin is injected, they quickly return to normal weight. Related to the carbohydrates-cause-weight-gain theory is the fact that insulin (stimulated by carb eating) blocks or inhibits the leptin signal to the brain. This condition allows people to continue eating even when their stomachs should be telling them they have attained enough energy.

Another interesting factor in the leptin scenario is that it instigates a signaling protein (VEGF) that is strongly associated with blood vessel health. Included is the capacity to reduce the inflammation that is associated with coronary plaque as well as plaque in the brain strongly suspected with the Parkinson's and Alzheimer's disease processes.

Two ways to promote healthy leptin activity are to reduce insulin through low-carb eating and engaging in high-intensity exercise. Remember that sugars and refined carbohydrates trigger the drive to continue eating them and that fats provide satiety. Less hunger and using stored fat for needed energy sounds pretty good. Hey, this plan might really work for you like it has for tens of thousands of others!

Increased Metabolic Rate

Metabolic rate refers to the speed of our metabolism—the rate at which our body uses energy or burns calories. The higher the metabolic rate, the faster we burn calories 24/7, when walking standing, exercising, and even sleeping and eating. It's a critical element related to any plan to lose weight (fat) and build/tone muscle. Ideally, we want to increase this rate so that we are efficiently burning the calories that will help us lose weight. This is another highly misunderstood area of physiology prevalent in the exercise/weight-loss arena. There is no reasonable debate about the conclusion that increased lean weight (especially muscle mass) increases metabolic rate. But believe it or not, some folks, who should know better, still don't understand that a higher muscle "weight" is almost always related to a positive state of fat control and should be treated as a separate issue from overall body weight. Skeletal muscles require much more energy for simple maintenance than either fat or bones, for example. Some organs, especially the brain, also have high levels of metabolic (calorie burning) demand. Having established that fact, stimulating muscle growth is still the best way to prevent metabolic slowdown during dietary weight reduction, aging, and any exercise regimen intended to "burn" more fat.

The underlying driving force of exercise is its capacity to alter metabolism. In simple terms, positively changing your metabolism involves becoming a fat burner instead of a fat storer. Because the body is naturally protective against metabolic change, that change must be powerfully driven. Depending on the muscle mass status of the individual, properly conducted high intensity exercise increases metabolism to burn more calories and provides strong resistance against normal aging and simple caloric reduction (diet) effects. When you simply decrease calories indiscriminately, it has been established that weight loss is composed of losing equal amounts of fat and muscle. That is NOT a good metabolic move unless you are more than 50 percent body fat—and that condition would be categorized as a state of morbid obesity.

Another reason for engaging in high intensity exercise while trying to reduce body fat is that exercising muscles burn calories at an elevated rate when compared to non-lean tissue. In simple terms, not only is resting metabolic rate enhanced, but also exercising metabolic rate is significantly increased. You burn more calories resting and exercising if you increase lean muscle tissue. It's a Win/Win/Lose fat situation!

Remember, burning a few hundred calories exercising won't hurt if it doesn't make you hungry and slow down your metabolism during recovery, but increasing calorie burning by 20-40 calories per hour, 24 hours a day, as a result of increased lean tissue activity can add up to create a considerable fat deficit, and I have observed and measured this consistently for many decades. Remember, the caveat that exercise (at lower levels of intensity) momentarily burns calories BUT the aftereffects of this type of activity are increased hunger and fatigue. Both of these responses work against long-term fat loss or in many cases produce inconsequential or minimal responses in the weight-loss battle.

Inflammation and Exercise

The role of inflammation in the human body is an extremely intricate, influential, and interesting component of function and health. Inflammation is basically the result of any imbalance in the chemical processes that are ongoing 24 hours a day in human metabolism. It is a prominent factor in the checks and balances system of dynamic health.

Here's a simple but relevant example. When we exercise, we "rock the boat" metabolically. Resting metabolism is fairly even-keeled in the long run in relatively healthy individuals. When something changes, like demanding higher levels of fueling for increased muscle action (exercise), the resting chemistry is upset and creates a reaction. That reaction can increase blood flow, deform tissue (stretch and compress), and cause a reaction called inflammation.

Human bodies evolved to respond to inflammation by adapting and instigating changes that would be more receptive to that stress the next time it might be encountered. In the case of exercise, the body responds in a healthy manner by increasing its capacity to engage in future muscular demands. There are a couple of "catches": The inflammation must be small enough not to cause irreversible damage, and there must be adequate time for the repair or response to come to fruition (completion). The analogy that I use to demonstrate this mechanism is the suntan: If you lie in the sun for a limited amount of time every other day, you can normally expect an adaptation of increased melanin (darker skin tone), because we have caused some degree of inflammation but not too much to cause tissue damage. If, however, you spend five hours a day, five days in a row, in the sun, you can expect a sunburn or sun poisoning, because the inflammation would have accumulated to such a high degree that it would be too great to induce healthy compensation.

Inflammation gets a bad rap because it is cited as the cause of many health problems and diseases, such as heart disease, diabetes, arthritis, and some forms of cancer. The body also uses inflammation to repair tissue and regrow effected tissue (usually to an elevated, more capable state). In other words, "micro damage" is fine, but "macro damage" is harmful. A common example of "micro" damage is the formation of a callous. When you use your hands repeatedly in sports or perhaps in physical labor, such as shoveling, you irritate the area of contact. That produces an inflammatory response: red, irritated, slightly tender skin. Given a few days to recover and then repeating the maneuver causes the eventual, protective adaptation of a callous.

However, if you repeatedly perform the same movement vigorously for hours at a time with little recovery allowed, the inflammation overwhelms the adaptive process and injury occurs or "macro damage." Interestingly, some foods can be categorized as "inflammatory," since many folks have an adverse response to their ingestion. Even when people are not allergic to (or not considered intolerant of) certain food groups like wheat, dairy, and simple sugars, these can be irritating to large numbers of people.

Intermittent inflammation is normal; constant inflammation is usually detrimental. For example, getting an upset stomach once in awhile from some spicy food can be overcome by the body's repair response (an intermittent inflammation). Muscle cells and nerve cells have an innate, "hardwired" repair (recovery and adaptation) mechanism that is activated by the stress of moderate, intermittent inflammation. But if the stomach is repeatedly irritated by certain foods, the inflammation can be overwhelming and cause significant tissue damage (constant inflammation).

In the specific instance of exercise, it is obvious that too much is counterproductive and exhausting. By the same token, exercise that causes no significant response or metabolic upheaval is nonproductive. Therefore, stresses and resulting inflammation must be orchestrated expertly to produce safe, consistent, and steady responses. In the realm of exercise, for example, if the session is exhausting and repeated before the body can healthily respond to the upheaval in our chemistry, inflammation will quickly halt any progress and, in some cases, reverse it. If, on the other hand, the disruption in our chemistry is significant enough to cause a subtle inflammatory response, the body will adapt upwardly if given an ample period in which to recuperate and respond. In fact, there is plenty of evidence that high intensity exercise, adroitly applied, can instigate a highly anti-inflammatory response.

It's not MAGIC.

It's not a SECRET.

It's a logical application of recognized science and basic human study data.

The modern lifestyle dilemma with inflammation is that it has evolved from a healing method for trauma encountered on an irregular basis (hunter/gatherer stresses, injuries, and so on) to a lower level constant state of irritation. If this vaguely detectable level of inflammation is left unchallenged by a counterbalancing physical response (higher intensity exercise, for example), it becomes degenerative and fosters ill health. For example, workplace stress (deadlines, arrogant supervisors, office politics) that exists constantly commonly wears on people at the point of organic inflammation, causing headaches, stomach problems, and so on. Left unchecked, these levels of inflammation become degenerative unless alleviated by behaviors like exercise, healthy diet, and good sleep patterns.

Exercise Grows Your Brain!

There is a clear link between physical fitness and mental performance, including memory, academic achievement, behavioral and social acclimatization, and cognitive function. By now, almost everyone understands that exercise is a SMaRT activity to do for a lifetime. It seems that the muscle system is much more significant in the scheme of overall health and function for many other systems, including brain function, than previously recognized.

Substantial, bona fide research has indicated generally that the brain requires significant physical activity to function optimally. Specifically, cognitive function, academic performance, memory, problem-solving, mood, stress, anxiety, ADHD, Alzheimer's, hormone flux, and the ravages of aging can be significantly improved through the proper application of simple exercise.

As in the case of many of the benefits of exercise, a simple review of evolutionary anthropology provides the logical explanation. Our human gene structure was developed by thousands of years of vigorous physical movement. The growth of the human brain was influenced by the ability to support about 10 miles of movement per day for extended periods of time: patience in hunting down prey for food, tact in designing strategies for hunting, and strength for short bursts of maximal physical efforts. It has been proposed that the large size of the human brain is directly correlated with supporting challenging muscle work—exercise and coordinated physical activity.

The human brain is primarily composed of an intricate, huge series of nerve connections: 100 BILLION brain cells, EACH with 1,000 connections. In spite of that capacity, I still find it hard to comprehend that number! In any case, just as I have traced the development of the physical exercise demands of genetically driven behavior, I will attempt to present the brain's developmental history.

Remember, the body works by sending signals. This concept is also applicable with brain function. The brain interprets and redirects the signals to drive immediate action and regulate functional capacities for future demands. In simple terms, the brain can react instantaneously when it is required and additionally "files" the information so that the appropriate systems can respond by adapting to that signal in the future.

In the case of a particular exercise, the muscles demand a certain recruitment of muscle fibers. Instantly, the brain—the master controller of the nervous system—signals muscle action and support from the cardiovascular, respiratory, and hormonal systems to accomplish the immediate task. That is called the acute response. As a result of all that exercise, a particular chemical "soup" is concocted. The "flavor" and subtleties of that situation are further interpreted by the brain in order to send longer term signals to all the systems involved. That set of signals instigates the changes that will occur in a healthy body response. We call these changes adaptations or "results."

Two major responses occur that involve the brain/exercise connection: First, the brain is intricately and substantially stimulated by the exercise action. It is coerced to respond quickly and strongly. As a result, the brain "grows"—literally, "growth factors" are driven. Second, as a result of this adaptation, the brain is now more capable of warding off degenerative processes associated with depression, anxiety, ADHD, Alzheimer's, Parkinson's disease, and a host of other brain-related disorders. Exercise has been unequivocally proven to stimulate the release of VEGF (vascular endothelial growth factor) and FGF-2 (fibroblast growth factor). These names mean nothing to the layman, but they are two powerful signaling proteins that induce the brain to grow new connections and nerve cells, thus increasing the vibrancy and resilience of the brain to function in a healthy, vigorous, youthful manner. Yes, "growing" the brain works just like "growing" muscles. This process allows both—muscles and brain—to function at a higher level of efficiency and capacity and carries a strong health protective component. "A sound mind in a healthy body" really applies in the case of SMaRT Exercise.

Back to human brain evolution. Our brains, as a direct response to physical exercise and activity, have developed into proportionately large and intricate organs. Without this multi-thousand-year stimulus process, our brains would NOT have developed nearly to the extent that they have. Brain scans have revealed that certain areas can actually grow and shrink just like muscles do. When the brain grows, it is reflective of a positive metabolic change in potential capacity. In simple terms, when the brain adds to the functional nerve volume, it is said to be in a healthier state. When it shrinks, conditions such as Alzheimer's and Parkinson's can be detected among other degenerative processes. In a number of cases, exercise has been directly responsible for this increase in brain volume and function. It just reinforces the concept that it is SMaRT to exercise!

Exercise of significant intensity reduces stress and instigates healthy brain chemistry, including managing stress disorders and anxiety. A Duke study had one group of depressed females take Prozac and the other matched group engaged in real, organized exercise. Both groups showed significant improvement, but the exercise group had no chemical side effects. Exercise also has a serious impact on academic performance and intelligence. In study after study, students who are more physically active achieve higher levels of academic competence. They also have fewer behavioral problems, less truancy, and higher rates of graduation and college attendance. The beneficial chemistry of exercise as it relates to brain health and function is undeniable, and for those of us who have passed the student phase of our lives, it might very well be more important than it was when we were younger.

A powerful connection exists between healthy, enhanced levels of circulation and an innumerable number of degenerative conditions, including basic aging. As nerve mass decreases, the function of that area of the brain is always compromised. This decrease is directly related to impaired circulation (blood flow) and depressed instigation of growth factors, both of which are consistently enhanced by serious exercise exposure. In fact, if applied in a responsible and expert manner, exercise and diet can prevent, reverse, and manage most of the degenerative diseases that plague modern man.

• • •

Hopefully, now you can understand how our bodies have been designed for survival and therefore actually function best when we perform high intensity exercise. The type of targeted exercise proposed by the SMaRT program affects how our body stores sugar, regulates insulin, and encourages our metabolism to burn fat. Even our brain benefits from regular physical activity. If one of your goals is to engage in exercise that drives many of the benefits that we are all looking for—fat burning, muscle building, health generating, and brain boosting—then high intensity muscle work properly applied goes a long way toward those aspirations. In the next chapter, we'll discover the troubling origins of the low-fat industry, why it is a large part of the reason so many people struggle with weight, and the real reason we *should* be eating more fat in our diets.

CHAPTER TWO

FAT IS SKINNY

By the mid 1980s the dye had been cast: Saturated fat and choles-terol were the heart-killing culprits. It was pronounced by "sci-ence," government, and media that the only way to ward off this impending doom was to cut back on fats and to run our hearts into better shape. The fitness boom and more "heart healthy" grains, fruits, and vegetables became the calling card for the reversal of our epidemic health problems.

The dissenters in the academic and clinical arenas were drowned out—and virtually shut out—of the process. However, some of us stuck to our guns and kept raising rather simple ques-tions. Why didn't the science add up to support the propagation of these theories? Why did replacing fat with sugar become a better metabolic solution for reversing fat-related disorders? Why was more and more exercise required to battle our bulge? What went wrong? Well, unfortunately, the research process was driven by money, with certain industries granting funds to promote their own agendas. The topper was when the McGovern Senate Commit-tee issued the Dietary Goals for the United States in 1977, demon-izing fat and professing that fats were damaging the health of our nation, and it was in the best interest of everyone if we cut down on this dastardly food type in general and saturated fats specifically.

Why was the perpetuation of this opinion so damaging? For one, the science was WRONG, and two, it was reported that even Marc Hedsted, a fervent "fat is deadly" advocate stated, "Practically nobody (scientists present at the hearings) was in favor of the McGovern recommendations." The movement generated a bandwagon of panic and fear of fat but was grounded in no real data or science. This move would change the "science" and recommended eating habits of an entire nation for decades.

Obesity has been around for centuries, but the recent significant escalation in the condition is certainly a legitimate cause for alarm. With all the advances in modern medicine, there is no pharmaceutical cure for it. Diabetes, also a recent epidemic condition, is poorly managed at best by drug intervention. Why have these conditions grown exponentially in the past 35 years?

Is there an answer? How do we handle these life-threatening problems? Well, we know what doesn't work as witnessed by what we've been doing. First, it would seem logical to direct efforts towards preventing or greatly reducing the *causes* of these conditions, rather than trying to "patch up" the symptoms after the fact. However, this is not to suggest that these problems can't be reversed once they occur. The calories in and calories out model that encompasses almost every plan to fight fat-related problems is organically flawed and overly simplistic. The composition of foods—carbs, proteins, fats—is much more relevant than the simple calculation of calories. The effect that the types of calories have on our metabolism is far more important than the simple number of calories they contain. As you will see in this chapter, fat can actually make you skinny—and it may be the most important nutrient you can consume to lose weight.

The Lipid Hypothesis: Bad Science!

If, as history indicates, something in our collective metabolic state has dramatically changed and threatened our health status, shouldn't we examine the possibilities? Shouldn't someone have been looking at the progression of fat-related disorders, such as obesity, diabetes, and metabolic syndrome? That seems SMaRT! Allowing the declining situation to continue unabated for more than 40 years and abiding by the same supposedly "healthy" low-fat diet philosophy, however, is *not* smart.

Examine the following history and allow common sense to determine if we have been deliberately misled or if some influential scientists and politicians have made some serious errors. "Science" reinforced by the American Heart Association, the American Dietetic Association, the US and British government health agencies, and many others told us to eat low-fat diets to reduce high cholesterol because they claimed that saturated fats caused blockage of coronary arteries and therefore caused heart attacks and strokes. Again, the "science" said to eat low fat, but based on what?

Well, in 1954, David Kritchevsky performed a study on rabbits, force feeding them a high-cholesterol diet. They developed plaque on their arteries (albeit different plaque than the human blockage type). That's part of the scientific basis of the "lipid hypothesis." I guess no one told anyone that rabbits are vegetarians whose livers can't metabolize cholesterol. Bad science!

In the 1960s, Ancel Keys supervised and published a six-nation nutritional analysis study indicating a correlation between eating animal fats and heart disease. When scrutinized a little more closely, the study originally included twenty-two nations and that data revealed an *opposite* tendency or *no effect* from eating higher fat diets. Unfortunately, this study was cited time and again as the "scientific" basis for low-fat eating. Bad science!

In 1977, the McGovern's senate select committee issued "dietary goals for the US." These goals advised a reduction of all fats, especially saturated fats, because of the relationship to "leading causes of death in the US." Opposing information provided by Dr. Fred Kummerow of the University of Illinois was excluded from the published information. Governmental propagation of bad science!

As a result of these recommendations, the United States Department of Agriculture constructed the following dietary guidelines, which continue to this day:

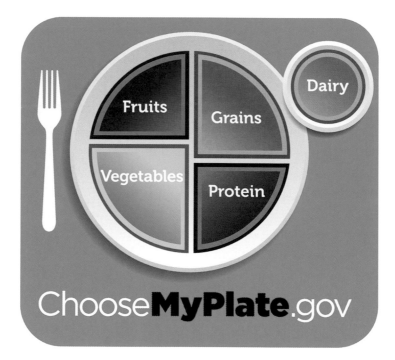

As you can see from this pie chart, we are officially told to structure our diets from a base of 75 percent carbohydrates. This is *exactly* why we have become a fatter, more diabetic, and sicker nation! The simple takeaway is this: Carbohydrates drive an elevated insulin response, which drives fat storage. What is the main problem with obesity and fat-related disorders? Fat storage gone awry.

Why We Should Have Known Better

Clinical evidence and published writings dealing with heart disease, cholesterol, and obesity treatment date back more than one hundred years. Before science strayed, the universal stance was that reducing carbohydrates and eating natural fats, sometimes only meat, was the customary, accepted medical treatment for combating obesity.

In 1907, Vil Stefansson went to live with the Arctic Inuits whose diet consisted of whale and seal meat and fatty fish. There were no fruits available and almost no edible vegetation. Despite this highly saturated, fat-oriented diet, the Inuits demonstrated no dietary problems like heart disease, diabetes, cancer, or obesity. "Science" frowned upon Stefansson's findings, attributing it to some genetic aberration—even though Stefansson himself thrived on this diet healthfully for a year while living with the Inuits. He also repeated this diet while in New York for a year, displaying the same health and vigor that he had noted on his journeys.

In 1939, Dr. Westin Price published his "Nutrition and Physical Degeneration," in which he described ten years of investigation of primitive populations and their dietary habits. He concluded that the primitive diets were principally high in fats, including meats, fish, and game with little in the way of fruits and vegetables. These populations were virtually free of degenerative diseases like cancer, heart disease, and diabetes. When "Western" diets, including sugars and refined carbohydrates, were introduced, the incidence of our modern diseases increased in a matter of a few generations.

The Maasai in Africa have been studied from the 1920s until the present, including the work of Dr. George Mann, indicating that their diet of meat, milk, and animal blood was constructed of a mainly saturated fat basis. The result was virtually no heart disease or obesity. When the Maasai move to urban settings and eat refined carbohydrates and sugars, their "immunity" to modern metabolic disorders disappears.

In India in 1967, Dr. Malhotra studied the people of Madras, along with the people in Punjab. The Punjabis ate 15 times the fat of the Madrasis and had 1/7 the rate of heart disease. A high-fat diet reduced heart disease by 86 percent!

In a number of national studies regarding high-fat diets, the intended outcomes demonizing fat actually revealed paradoxical results. The more fat that was consumed, the less problematic was heart disease, obesity, and diabetes. In fact, here is a list of some of the national studies that provided unexpected results: The French Paradox, The Alpine Paradox, The Greek Paradox, The Spanish Paradox, The Northern Ireland Paradox, The Israeli Paradox, The Indian Paradox, and The Japanese Paradox. Paradox? Obviously not!

Still government science and health science continue to demonize high-fat diets. We're told that to eat "healthy," we must minimize fat intake, especially saturated fat. As you will see, this is a huge mistake, and our bodies need fat as a primary fuel source to function at their best.

Fat Literally Keeps Us Alive

We can store hundreds of thousands of fat calories, and we can store 1,000 to 2,000 calories of carbohydrates. Let's take an educated guess as to which fuel source—fat or carbs—was the main sustainer of evolving human life? Fat. It was and *is* the primary fuel upon which the healthy human body depends.

Fat is the preferred fuel for keeping our bodies consistently functioning at a healthy energy level. We obviously have a large capacity to store fat, and this trait has kept us alive through thick and thin (literally). Remember, we had fuel available in sporadic intervals for the first two million plus years of existence. For that reason, the survivors of human development have an "ingrained" or genetic tendency to use only the fat necessary to support metabolic activity. The rest is stored for times of scarcity.

Since the inception of the modern "healthy eating" paradigm, our sugar consumption has increased by more than 30 pounds annually since 1960! If we have limited healthy sugar storage capacities as human animals, what happens when we consistently inundate our systems with that fuel source?

We get fat.

We also get sick.

Those directly related sicknesses include obesity, diabetes, many forms of cancer, arthritis, and a myriad of other inflammatory disorders. As strange as it might appear upon initial observation, fat-related disorders are substantially instigated by the inability to healthily partition sugar as either circulating or stored fuel.

Sugar—the Real Culprit in Making Us Fat

If we can assume that a simple calories in to calories out model is not truly representative of the "fattening" process, then perhaps we can find a rational explanation. Certainly, our genetic blueprint has much to do with our body composition but, by the same token, it can't explain the recent fattening of America (or the rest of the "developed" world). So something different has been occurring and at a rapid pace. Genes don't change in 40 years and probably not even in 400 or 1,000 years. That causal difference has to be behavioral.

We have to be doing something drastically different than we were 40-50 years ago. In fact, some people have indicated that such an abrupt change must be related to a toxin—a poison that our collective bodies can't overcome. Some believe that poison is fructose.

Fructose is the sugar found primarily in fruits and, coincidently, the major component in high-fructose corn syrup. Imagine the maple syrup you put on your pancakes in the morning that makes them taste extra delicious. Now imagine putting that syrup on almost *everything* you eat. Your Mom would say, "Don't do that. It will make you sick." Well, high fructose corn syrup has been added to all manufactured bread products, prepared food, frozen foods, and more—it is found in virtually every bread-related product in every supermarket. All this sugar in all of our foods is literally making us sick. More data has accumulated in recent years, leading us to believe that fructose can be an unusually toxic form of sugar. Included in those accusations is the theory that fructose actually starts the metabolic ball rolling in the wrong direction for many people. Once the body is inundated with fructose, more and more carbohydrates become inflammatory as our sensitivity becomes heightened and more problematic.

One last note on fructose: It can only be metabolized in the liver—and much of that process turns this sugar directly into fat. That's right: Sugar turns into fat in a process called "de novo lipogenisis," which means making new fat. So even if you think you're eating a high-carb, *low-fat* diet, and it contains any highly processed foods and/or multiple servings of fruit products, you're more than likely eating a high-carb, *high-fat* diet—and that's a really bad plan.

So what is the takeaway from all of this history and science of eating? Simply this: In order to maintain a healthy weight or to start the process of losing fat, you need to cut down significantly on carbohydrates, especially sugars and refined carbohydrates like pasta, cereals, and cookies.

Eat Fat to Lose Fat

If we dramatically reduce carbohydrates—especially sugars and refined carbs—with what do we replace all of those calories that we actually need? The only remaining possibilities are either protein or fats. We certainly need protein to maintain lean tissue and build all manner of tissues and organ cells. However, there is a limit to the amount or percentage of protein that we can utilize effectively in our diets without running into some overload problems. After initial protein levels are met, the inclusion of healthy fats is the most efficient way to lose weight and enhance health. The upside of protein intake is that, under normal circumstances, the body uses protein initially to maintain and regain tissue that structures cells. In simple terms, about 60 to 100 grams of protein is used up for tissue construction projects before it is even considered as a fuel source. So, in a way, protein has a "free calorie" status to a certain extent when it comes to fat storage or accumulation problems.

Fats provide even more satiety than protein, and protein beyond the point of sufficiency can instigate some insulin response. My years of clinical experience have demonstrated that between one-half and one gram of protein per pound of lean body weight usually works well for most. (Check your lean body weight as calculated by your body composition charts in chapter four.) As a result, we're left with the healthy choice of our predominant food source: Fat.

An interesting note on the maintenance of fat loss described as long-term fat loss: This is perhaps more elusive than losing weight in the first place. How many of us have experienced the loss of weight only to have it return time and again? In 1956, two British researchers, Alan Kekwick and Gaston Pawan, put obese subjects on 1,000 calorie per day diets. They split the group into balanced (higher level carbohydrate), high protein (90 percent protein), and high fat (90 percent fat). The carbohydrate subjects actually began to *gain* weight (even on only 1,000 calories per day). The high-protein dieters steadily lost weight. But the high-fat subjects lost more weight, more rapidly than the others.

Perhaps even more interesting, when the subjects were fed a 2,600 calorie, high-fat diet, they continued to lose weight. In conclusion, these same people who were actually gaining weight on a 1,000 calorie per day, carbohydrate inclusive diet started losing weight on a 2,600 calorie per day, high-fat diet—additional, compelling evidence that a calorie is certainly NOT a calorie!

Back to fat facts: Fats have to be available in the form of fatty acids to be actively used for fuel. The rest of fat is stored in the form of triglycerides. When more fatty acids are circulating than can be used for imminent fueling, they return to storage or accumulate in the bloodstream as triglycerides. In fact, fat cycles in and out of storage (triglyceride) and usage (fatty acids) continuously in the body. Cholesterol is over-hyped as a "bad blood lipid," but triglycerides are the real blood fat culprits (cholesterol isn't really even technically a fat). High triglyceride levels are directly correlated with a myriad of health problems. The simple takeaway from this information is that anything that drives fat into triglyceride form also drives fat "storage."

Triglycerides (technically triglycerol) are formed because fats (fatty acids) don't store readily on their own (singularly). They need a little help to be packaged better for optimal storage. The eating of carbohydrates produces a by-product molecule called alpha glycerol phosphate, which conveniently offers the "phosphate" part of it to join with three fat molecules (fatty acids) to form "tri" (three fatty acids) and a "glyceride" (the "glycerol" part of the alpha glycerol phosphate). Some of the triglycerides in our fat come directly from eating fat, but the rest come from eating carbohydrates. This means it's the carbohydrates that drive the formation and storage of triglyceride that are the bad fats in excess.

Conversely, anything that drives fatty acid release drives fat utilization (burning). The right kind of eating (lower carbs) and exercise (higher intensity) are a potent combination for reducing triglycerides when they are problematic and keeping their buildup at a healthy level of storage. When the body needs stored fat to provide and supplement fuel needs, it has to break down (separate) the fatty acids from the glycerol to be transported out of storage. Eating low-carb based foods allows this release and use of stored fat to occur more readily, and high intensity exercise triggers an adrenaline response that demands that the fat stored as triglyceride become ready for backup fuel. It is therefore broken down and drawn out of storage. That's a very GOOD thing for reducing stored fat!

Fat Storage

Remember, as a species, humans can only survive if we have energy available to fuel our organs. Therefore, we stash fuel when we can in order to have some reserves. A certain level of fuel storage in the form of fat and sugar is healthy.

The modern-day energy or fuel dilemma really results from the body's problem with partitioning that fuel when it is available in excess. Where does the body put it? The simple answer is "where it belongs." In fact, the healthiest place for excess energy to be stored is probably in fat cells, where it does the least amount of harm. People who have energy storage problems and still retain normal body fat levels often present more severe metabolic problems than those who are overweight or obese. This might sound confusing, but here's an explanation: When fat can not be used for immediate fueling purposes, it has to be stored or placed somewhere. The healthiest selection for that storage place is in fat cells. They have evolved to handle this task of storage in their specific manner. If, however, these cells do NOT take on their genetic responsibilities, the fat must go somewhere else. These other places are not designed to handle the fat that they must now deal with, and they eventually break down from the intrusion and overload (liver, heart, blood vessels, and so on). Again, excess energy storage, the availability of too much energy for healthy storage and reserve, seems to be at the root of many of our metabolic problems. In conclusion, many people who do not express their metabolic dysfunction (disease) by becoming fat or obese can suffer severe health consequences as a result of misplaced energy storage.

Reserved energy can be healthily stored as triglyceride in fat cells either under the skin or to a much lesser extent in between or inside organs. However the deposit of "belly fat," called "visceral" fat, is strongly associated with greatly increased diabetes, cardiac risk, and severely compromised health. Generally, excess fat deposits above the waist in the belly area are more than likely representative of metabolic disease. That's why in younger (premenopausal) women, the "pear" shape of fat deposit (below the waist) is much less related to disease risk than the predominantly male "apple" shape, with fat being distributed in a round belly (beer gut) configuration. Since excess carbohydrate consumption leads to excess levels of fat being driven into storage then it is the carbohydrate problem that is most logically connected to the "beer belly" syndrome.

Metabolically induced fat storage (fat stored in excess due to compromised health) is a marker directly associated with a number of our most prevalent health problems, including obesity, overweight, syndrome x, diabetes, arthritis, heart disease, some forms of cancer, auto-immune diseases, and more. So our challenge is to understand why this ever-growing fat accumulation is happening and how we can best address and reverse this situation. If one were to analyze the epidemic rate of fat-related disorders historically, we need to try to understand the relationship between increased sugar (carbohydrate) consumption and its influence on eventual fat storage. One important note: Much of the popular weight loss eating advice includes reducing fat "and" sugar consumption. These two macronutrients (fat and carbohydrates) are composed very differently and trigger hugely divergent metabolic pathways regarding fat storage.

Sugar is stored in the muscles and the liver. Our capacity to store sugar healthfully is limited. In an average-sized man, there is about a 1600 calorie storage capacity (75 percent in the muscles and 25 percent in the liver). That's about one day's worth of energy. Needless to say, one day's worth of energy reserve would not have sustained life during even a short time of food deprivation. The body's answer to this problem is long-term and higher-capacity energy storage in the form of fat. This is an important point to remember when we talk about fuel "preference" both in eating and in utilization. Our diets and our fuel preference should healthily revolve around fat.

Why Fat Gets a Bad Rap

We have been indoctrinated into thinking that fat is unhealthy and that saturated fat causes heart disease. That is simply false! It is extremely difficult to replace widely perpetuated misinformation with contradictory, albeit true, facts. It is hard for most to accept that fats don't make us fat. Carbohydrates do. Many people assume that the more saturated fat they eat, the more it will wind up in their bloodstream. False. This simply doesn't happen. The same holds true for cholesterol consumption. In fact, people with high cholesterol levels will decrease the production of cholesterol by the liver if they eat higher levels of cholesterol. The body tries to "even it out."

Here are some more "fat facts":

- **Fact:** The majority of fatty acids in cholesterol are unsaturated.

- **Fact:** High carbohydrate consumption will drive the storage of fat much more readily than eating fat.

- **Fact:** Eating a high-fat diet will drive fat usage and release more fat than any other arrangement of nutrient composition. *Eat fat to burn fat.*

In a simple study conducted by Cassandra Forsythe at the University of Connecticut, twenty people ate a low-fat diet and twenty people ate a high-fat diet for 12 weeks. When blood fats were measured, the low-fat group had lowered blood lipids or fat by 19 percent and the high-fat group had lowered blood lipids by 51 percent!

In my 40-plus year clinical practice, I see a phenomenon repeated over and over again. People are afraid of eating fats and, as a result, they are left with a dilemma. Unless you choose to eat from the protein category only high-protein foods low in fat, like egg whites, skim milk, lean meats,poultry, and fish, you don't have many other low-fat options. Since it should be understood that fats are the body's preferred fuel for promoting stored fat release and usage, they should not be frowned upon when selecting food choices for healthy weight loss. When I have lunch at my golf club, I tell the waitresses to fix my burger without a bun but with added Swiss cheese, bacon, and grilled onions. I remind them that I'm trying to get more fat into my diet. At first they think I'm joking, but over time I explain why this is the best way to ensure a low body fat. Now they call it a "Dr. Bo burger."

The Top Ten Reasons Fat Is Healthy

Remember that the problem with fat is not in eating it. It's in what our body chemistry "tells" us what to do with foods that create excesses in energy. In simple terms, do we store fat or do we utilize it as our primary source of healthy fueling? That's called fuel "partitioning." We can direct our "fuel partitioning" by reducing sugar and refined carbohydrate consumption, increasing our "good" fat intake, and assuring that our protein intake is sufficient to support vigorous muscle activity and tissue repair and rebuilding.

So now we have established that eating fat is the healthy option. Here's why:

1. It's the primary energy source our genes relied on to prosper as a developing species. In fact, without the specific fats derived from animals, our brains couldn't have grown to the advanced levels they have. Interestingly, human milk contains fatty acids that cow's milk does not. That is one reason why a cow's brain is about 2 percent (relatively) the size of a human's.

2. It provides the highest level of satiety. Fat doesn't instigate blood sugar fluctuations. It keeps our energy supply consistent with fewer dips and cravings. It simply makes sense when you're trying to reduce body fat that decreasing hunger will be an enormous help in achieving real weight-loss results. Less hunger equals more diet success. SMaRT!

3. Fat is necessary for maintaining lean body mass. In study after study, the findings reinforce the concept that higher fat diets reduce stored body fat. In fact, in a Swedish study performed at Gothenburg University, the findings revealed in a study of four-year-olds comparing average weight children and obese children eating the same caloric levels, that the obese children eating the same diet had essential nutrient deficiencies in vitamin D, essential fatty acids, and iron while the average weight children did not. This simply demonstrates the possible effect of obesity on normal fat metabolism and body composition.

4. Low-fat diets simply don't work, as observed by Dr. Walter Willet of Harvard University. In the US from 1978 to 1990, fat intake fell 11 percent, caloric intake fell almost 100 calories per day, the percentage of the population eating low-calorie (usually "low-fat") foods rose from 19 percent to 76 percent, and the overweight population increased by 31 percent!

5. If you're worried about high cholesterol and heart disease resulting from a high-fat diet, Stop worrying! Cholesterol profiles actually IMPROVE on high-fat, low-carbohydrate diets. Many studies reinforce this position, including a study published in 2004 in *The Journal of the American College of Nutrition.*

6. Contrary to what the government or nutrition "experts" may advise, "good fats" are actually the natural ones (animal and coconut), primarily saturated and monosaturated (olive, coconut, and sesame oil and nuts). The "bad" fats are the polyunsaturates (vegetable oils and margarines). Butter, seriously demonized by the low-fat zealots (including the government "nutritionists") is comprised of 30 percent monounsaturated fat, 50 percent saturated, and 15 percent medium-saturated fat. Butter inhibits growth of toxic fungi and contains fatty acids that disable viruses and that are also are anti-infective and anti-carcinogenic. Sounds healthy to me!

7. Omega-3 and omega-6 fats are beneficial in specific forms and proportions. The best sources of these fats are cod liver, flax oils, and egg yolks. The healthy ratio of omega-6 to omega-3 should be about 2 to 1. Unfortunately, our diets include many more omega-6 fatty acids than we need. That disrupts the balance between the anti-inflammatory omega-3s and inflammatory omega-6s. If people do not eat a lot of these foods that are good sources of omega fats, I would suggest to most of them that they take omega-3 and 6 supplements.

8. In the mid 1980s, Mary Enig, a nutritionist and researcher, warned that "trans" fats were harmful to our health. The government and scientific community ignored and excluded

her work. Thirty years later, all agreed that trans fats should be outlawed. We were told to avoid anything that includes "trans" fats, even though the government tells us that saturated fats are just as harmful. This is simply misinformation and compromises your health!

9. Your brain, nerves, and endocrine (hormone) systems all thrive on animal fats for optimal function.

10. Remember, animal fats are *not* totally composed of saturated fats as we are led to believe. For example, beef fat is 54 percent unsaturated, lard is 60 percent unsaturated, and chicken fat is 70 percent unsaturated.

• • •

The information in this chapter has hopefully explained why our diets should healthily revolve around fat—and have for millions of years. Low-fat diets simply don't work because they ultimately result in eating too many carbohydrates. It's not about calories; it's about chemistry and how our body uses certain foods for fuel. Sugar is the real cause of our declining health and growing obesity. Clearly, there is a lot of confusion, misinformation, and bad science regarding what we should be eating to lose weight, and as you'll see in the next chapter, there is also just as much confusion about how to properly exercise to reduce body fat.

CHAPTER THREE

EXERCISE, ACTIVITY, AND "FAT BURNING"

People are often confused about using exercise to reduce body fat, but diet alone won't turn on your body's signaling for optimal fat-burning. However, "all exercise is not created equally," and there is a major difference between exercise and activity. "Exercise" is a poorly defined term in popular as well as scientific literature and is about as clearly defined as using the term "medicine" to describe any and all pharmaceutical products. Many types of exercise result in producing an aftereffect that makes you tired and hungry but have no real impact on significant fat reduction. Contrary to often-cited "facts," aerobic exercise programs have been repeatedly studied and proven to be an inefficient method to achieve weight loss. However, there are other, more strategic, types of exercise that encourage your body to burn more fat, such as properly constructed resistance training, and we'll explore why these work.

This chapter will explain the different types of muscle fibers, and how activating the right fibers will drive an adrenaline response in your body that supports fat burning. Most people want to lose fat and increase muscle mass, bone mass, and metabolic rate and improve health and appearance. Fortunately, most of these goals can be approached in a safe, simple, and efficient manner. Exercise and activity—each a separate and distinct discipline— can be constructed to best instigate healthy, beneficial metabolic responses.

Why Diet Alone Isn't Sufficient

Diet is a critical part of any fat-burning program, and in the last chapter we discovered why it's better to consume fat than carbohydrates in order to reduce insulin resistance and drive fat out of storage. However, many people mistakenly believe that if they change their diets, they will lose the unwanted fat, even if they don't engage in any form of exercise. While changing your diet may certainly help—as long as you are not following a low-calorie, low-fat model—there are so many benefits to high intensity exercise that a change in diet alone can't provide. The following list reveals the extraordinary advantages of exercise.

Exercise Can/Diet Can't:

- **Increase your metabolism:** For all intents and purposes, exercise is a much more powerful driver of metabolic rate increase (higher rate of calorie burning) than diet intervention. By the simple mechanism of instigating increased muscle mass, metabolic rate is consistently enhanced.

- **Increase cardiovascular function:** While losing a large amount of weight by dieting can help cardiovascular performance, such as running, a high intensity exercise DEMANDS that the heart and blood vessels increase their functional capacity (pumping and delivering oxygen rich blood). The heart and blood vessels simply become "better" at their jobs.

- **Acutely change brain chemistry:** There is little debate that eating a low-carbohydrate diet reduces the likelihood of plaque forming on the brain and causes less free radical formation (bad stuff). However, exercise, even at lower levels of intensity, has been strongly associated with enhanced cognitive function and increased levels of neurotransmitters (good stuff). The logical assumption that I make is that since higher intensity exercise produces higher levels of "growth factors" (proteins that drive cell growth) in the body than previous levels, this means the higher levels of brain-related, "scientifically acronymed" growth factors (BNDF, NGF and IGF-1, for example) are also stimulated with this increased intensity.

- **Magnify fat release:** Traditional dieting (caloric and fat-reducing plans) can certainly lead to weight reduction, but carbohydrate reduction usually leads to a better ratio of fat loss to weight loss. However, neither example of caloric food manipulation can achieve the rate and level that the normal, healthy response to high intensity exercise can by burning the fat "candle" at both ends. Explanation: High intensity exercise (like SMaRT) drives fat out of storage to become a source of backup fuel during and after the exercise session. It also promotes the building of lean mass (muscle and bone), while also raising the metabolic (fat burning) rate 24/7.

- **Increase growth factors (these make cells regenerate to keep you looking young):** As mentioned before, exercise can promote the secretion of growth factors, which are simply proteins that signal youthful rates of cell regeneration and turnover. Diet can, at best, create a slight advantage in which this process might be accomplished. Again, exercise is a significantly more powerful tool for going in this direction.

- **Build muscle and bone:** Some courses of dietary intervention can SUPPORT muscle growth and reduce rate of bone loss, but, again, only intense levels of exercise can PROMOTE the actual growth of muscle and bone so critical to increased fat burning and youthful, vigorous physical function.

- **Produce heat shock proteins and hormone sensitive lipase:** A little bit technical but perhaps interesting is this fact: When body heat is raised, including during adrenaline surges, "signaling proteins" called HSPs (Heat Shock Proteins) are generated. These proteins signal powerful immune system levels of protection. Another common response to high intensity exercise promotes the secretion of an effective fat releaser (enzyme) called HSL (Hormone Sensitive Lipase). The presence of this protein (enzyme) triggers fat burning and stalls fat storage. There is nothing in the dietary arsenal that can match these effects.

- **Tax fight or flight fibers (makes cells more able to use fat):** Unless you eat in a scary restaurant (like the one in the *Godfather*), you will never tax your fight or flight muscle fibers as a result of eating. However, once again, exercise at higher intensity does, in fact, call upon our fight and flight muscle fibers, creating a metabolic milieu (chemical soup) that drives significant fat release from storage and provides excess energy and fat burning for some time after the exercise.

If you want to turn your body into a fat-burning machine, you must incorporate exercise into your weight-loss program. Being active is incredibly important for your overall wellness, but activity alone will not produce the benefits of a more formal, calculated exercise regimen.

Exercise versus "Activity"

We are constantly being told that if we are active, we will lose weight. But there is a huge difference between being active and engaging in the types of exercise that will actually reap the best results. Activity has become associated with anything from planting tomatoes or strolling through the mall to training for a triathlon. Exercise should be considered a separate entity from "activity." Physical activity is certainly beneficial, and in many cases enjoyable, but it simply does NOT have the same metabolic (fat burning) effect as targeted exercise that manipulates your muscle fibers in a specific way for productive weight loss (more on this later).

Activity is still important, and you should strive to incorporate activity into your lifestyle in order to counteract sedentary behavior. Many of us sit for hours at a time in front of computers, because in today's modern society most of us work in offices. In the Stone Age, sedentary behavior meant death. If you couldn't keep up with the pack, you couldn't avoid predators, get to food sources, and so on. You literally died. Today, sedentary behavior can still kill us, but it occurs more slowly from degenerative diseases. Sedentary behavior can most easily be described as lacking movement for extended periods of time. In my recent association with studies on the subject with Arizona State University, it has been noted that sitting is an unusually negative posture in regard to health risks of sedentary behavior.

Sitting (which most modern business folks do) often revolves around not moving and also positions the body at a number of right angles (hips, knees, ankles) that place the body into tendencies of poor circulatory flow. Think of a hose (or blood vessel) bent at right angles in three places and not moving out of that position. How would you assume the water flow would be in that hose? Pretty inadequate. The posture of sitting related to blood flow is just like a bent hose. That is a "Dr. Ben" observation that I have not seen in any literature. Activity is necessary for muscle stimulation. If your daily routine includes sitting for extended periods of time, get up and move around (stretch, walk, and so on) every 90 minutes or so for two or three minutes.

So we know it's important to be active, but what type of *exercise* is best? I've been asked this question thousands of times. My answer is "the one you'll actually do." In all seriousness, the best exercise is the one that will help you lose fat, increase muscle and bone mass, and maintain your health, and I have been studying this for years in order to create the most efficient, effective program.

As we noted in chapter one, human physiology evolved to support intermittent, vigorous activity. That said, the belief that "the more exercise you do, the better it is for you," is simply not true and unfortunately this often discourages people from exercising because it makes exercise seem more difficult and unattainable. In Neolithic times, humans had to exert a huge amount of energy a few times a week. However, if they had to do this every single day, they would have quickly become so exhausted that they would have become easy prey (literally). So, you see, more is not always better.

Since our modern lifestyle presents a different set of activity demands and food availability, we need to adjust our habits accordingly. The body works by sending signals from system to system, organ to organ, and cell to cell through our behavior. Therefore, we want to engage in exercises that send the appropriate signals—the ones that will give us the best results. In order to *change* our physical status, we have to do something different. Because activity is less structured and more random and intermittent than regular exercise, it's often not sufficiently taxing and doesn't drive the changes that will readily help you lose body fat.

Unfortunately, we are often given the wrong prescription. Here's a perfect example. Let's say you go to your doctor for a routine physical and he tells you that you have to lose weight. He reiterates that it's not healthy and you run the risk of early, serious development of obesity, heart disease, diabetes, and a host of other degenerative conditions. He's right. Next, he tells you that he wants you to reduce calories, limit fat intake, and start a walking program. There is one serious problem with this advice: It doesn't work. It if did, there would be a lot more lean, healthy people walking around. Exercise requires that muscles work. Engaging our muscles the right way positively impacts many other systems in our bodies: cardiovascular, respiratory, endocrine, nervous, skeletal, and so on.

Why Aerobic Exercise Doesn't Work
for Weight Loss

As a result of decades of indoctrination by media and, to an extent, the "assumed science" about exercising, many people believe that cardio activities like running, step aerobics, or spin class are the best way to burn fat and lose weight—and the longer the duration, the better. Not only is this not the case; it actually represents misinformation supporting an inefficient form of exercise. Why is "fat burning" aerobic exercise not correlated to successful fat loss? It's because aerobic exercise is actually "fat diverting," while anaerobic exercise, such as resistance training, is sugar burning but "fat drawing" in nature, meaning that it draws your fat out of storage.

One of the lies we've been told is that aerobic exercise burns fat by increasing our metabolism, but the opposite is true. After this type of exercise, we have *less* energy circulating in our system (since we "borrowed" the fat from our body's circulation system to support this activity.). So our body has two choices: Either it slows down or we become hungry to compensate for that lost energy. When we're hungry and tired, we eat more and do less. Aerobic exercise uses fat in circulation, causing a deficit and depleting our energy because fat is no longer going at the normal rate to our heart and lungs and other organs and tissues that use fat as their energy source.

Anaerobic exercise, instead, is the best type of exercise for real fat burning because it fools our bodies into an adrenaline response, which will get more "emergency" energy circulating and draw fat out of storage. What many people don't realize is that this type of anaerobic exercise also achieves substantial aerobic and cardio benefits, increasing functional heart efficiency.

In fact, we conducted a study to compare the outcomes of a traditional cardiovascular exercise program to those of a slow resistance training program. Ninety adults were randomly selected to engage in a five-week program of exercise. One group performed a twice weekly, 15 minute session, slow resistance training program, and the other group performed and averaged three hours and fifteen minutes of weekly standard cardiovascular or "aerobic" exercise. We measured the body composition, cardio-respiratory endurance, upper body strength, lower body strength, trunk flexibility, blood pressure, and heart rate both before and after treatment. Results revealed that the resistance training group significantly exceeded the cardio group in measurements of improved body composition (increased lean tissue and decreased fat content), cardiorespiratory endurance, upper and lower body strength, trunk flexibility, and decreased resting blood pressure and heart rate. Our study indicated that the average participant using the resistance training program lost ten pounds of body fat and increased lean tissue by eight pounds. The cardio group gained one pound of muscle and lost one pound of fat. Cardiovascular exercise alone does *not* burn fat.

Traditionally, exercise has been broken down into two categories: aerobic or endurance training and anaerobic or strength training. But a more accurate and applicable breakdown would be to examine the local and global exercise effects and responses. When we perform an exercise, we are usually creating a significant demand for energy within a set group of muscles. These are the "local" areas of muscle work, such as biceps, quadriceps, and so on. However, this local demand triggers a "global" or full body systems support response, so our heart rate and breathing rate may increase, changes in enzyme levels occur, and all manner of signaling proteins are generated. These are some of the global or metabolic responses to the local muscle work.

Maximum Fat Burning

With regard to fat burning, the two most important and applicable behavioral factors are exercise and diet. The pertinent question is what kind of exercise and what type of diet? The answer is: those that increase metabolism. In other words, what happens chemically during and as a result of a specific exercise or diet application? Remember, the body's cells and organs "talk" to each other through a series of chemical signals. Our exercise and eating are most productively manipulated by controlling and directing the chemical "signals" that they send. We can do this best through combining high intensity exercise with a controlled carbohydrate diet.

The rationale for controlling carbohydrates in the diet is in the "message" or effect it signals on insulin production, as discussed in chapter 2. Only carbohydrates trigger an immediate and significant release of insulin. Fats have no effect on insulin, and proteins have a delayed, vague effect (since they also trigger an equivalent response to the opposite acting hormone, glucagon). Next, if drawing fat out of storage is the objective of our exercise efforts, two simple points must be made: One is that aerobic, steady-state exercise does not and has not historically signaled support of that goal; and the second is that adrenaline signals the immediate release of free fatty acids from their storage form (triglycerides) to reinforce the emergency demand of an unusual physical circumstance. That's what high intensity muscle demand does. It signals an impending emergency. By controlling this signaling mechanism, high intensity exercise manipulates glycogen depletion and fat utilization in a similar, more exaggerated manner than carbohydrate restriction does. Together, they create a synergistically powerful metabolic force.

Whereas steady state aerobic exercise creates a deficit of post-exercise energy, since it has been drawn upon during the event, high intensity anaerobic exercise creates an "overshoot" of available energy, unless the bout of exercise is excessive or exhaustively traumatic. By specifically organizing and controlling how we exercise our muscles, we can guide our metabolisms toward the fat-burning mode and our muscles to force fat out of storage and drive protein towards the increase in muscle activity and mass. This combination of events promotes a leaner, healthier body composition: less fat, more muscle. Body composition is defined as the percentage of body tissue comprised of lean (muscle and bone) and fat tissue. This measurement has been, in my practice, a valuable objective tool for assessing exercise and diet productivity.

In the case of the overwhelming majority of individuals, the goal of exercise and diet plans is to reduce body fat and increase, or at least maintain, lean tissue. Lean tissue (bone and muscle) is sometimes overlooked in the blinders of a fat reduction program. Sure, losing fat is a good thing, but building lean tissue means increasing calories burned in resting and exercising states and building bone activity. Both of these mechanisms are vital in "signaling" positive health status.

Certain types of exercise increase your metabolism and build muscle. For many, building muscle is a much more subtle process than that sought after by elite athletes and certainly bodybuilders, but it requires a similar signaling. A more active muscle system simply indicates a more vibrant, youthful status of chemical processing than that same muscle system (yours) resulting from little extraordinary stimulus. In simple terms, the stimulus of high intensity exercise demands that our muscle systems must be working at a higher level of turnover and replenishment (like it does more "naturally" when we're young). In other words, you have to physically *do* something significant in order to initiate a continuously active muscle metabolism. Remember—your body, left to its own devices, wants to maintain the status quo (homeostasis). Collectively, we, as folks trying to regain or attain a lean body composition, want to CHANGE the status quo until we reach our desired goals.

With regard to fat burning, let's begin with the simple formula that most people think controls fat "burning" or loss. Eat fewer calories (IN) and exercise more calories (OUT) or "in one end and out the other," so to speak. It doesn't work! It's NOT the way the human body was designed. We are not simple mechanical, robotic mechanisms. We are metabolic (chemically-driven) creatures. Don't buy this explanation? How can the average woman gain four to five pounds in three days every month? Did she unconsciously eat an additional 14,000 to 17,000 calories in those three days? A week later when she loses the weight, did she also unconsciously run or walk an extra 140 to 170 miles? Those are examples of how utterly silly a simple thermodynamic (calories IN/ calories OUT) model of energy (calorie) balance really is.

To instigate real fat burning, you need to engage in exercise that taxes your system. This varies, depending upon how fit you are. Our goal is to manipulate the muscles so that they reach a threshold level. My threshold example: When you push a rock to the edge of a sheer cliff and push it over the edge, once it begins to fall, you no longer have to do anything. It's the same with your muscles: Once you stimulate all muscle fiber types to their threshold levels, you can rest and your body will continue to burn fat and continue the muscle-building process. What does this mean? Well, our muscles have different types of fibers that our body utilizes, depending upon whether we need them for endurance or strength, and the best form of exercise engages all of our muscle fibers at once, as I will explain in more detail in the next section.

Types of Muscle Fibers

To better understand exactly why anaerobic exercise burns fat, it helps to understand how our muscle fibers work. Muscle fibers were initially categorized as "red" or "white" because the staining techniques originally utilized discerned only the gross differences between capillary rich (red)—or what is known as "slow twitch"—and capillary sparse (white) known as "fast twitch." More advanced lab techniques further distinguished muscles into four "fiber types": Type I, Type II a, Type II ab, and Type II b. Type I fibers are still called "slow twitch" fibers and all Type II fibers are called "fast twitch" fibers. The description of skeletal muscle fiber types refers to the range of fatigue, or how fast they get tired. All skeletal muscles are composed, to some degree, of all of these four subtypes. When we are simply hanging out and walking around, we use our Type I muscle fibers, which have the most endurance—they are slow to get tired—but little strength. When we need progressively more strength to perform an activity, we call upon the Type II fibers, which can handle more strenuous activity but for shorter periods of time, as they tire out more quickly (than the Type I's). Our muscles follow a pattern of recruitment from the weakest to the strongest: Type I to Type II a to Type II ab and finally to Type II b.

Muscle fibers will grow to attain more strength capacity or potential. The scientific word for that growth is "hypertrophy." However, if certain fiber types can't handle a load imposed upon them, they will—in order—call upon the next, stronger fiber type to accomplish the desired task. It's like the gears on a bike. For simply cruising around, first gear is fine. But when you need to pedal up a hill, you need to switch to a higher gear. It's the same with your muscles—you won't be able to do it for long, but I want you to get to that higher gear or muscle fiber type and drive the adrenaline response in your body to change the chemistry or metabolism that will induce fat burning. That means that Type I fibers will try as hard as they can but will have to call upon Type II fibers if they can't handle the load by themselves. They will keep trying and stay "turned on" during progressively more demanding, or heavier, loads. The weaker, lower strata, slower twitch fibers really don't have to grow or hypertrophy to any great extent if they can call upon the next readily available "stronger" muscle fiber type. In fact, slow twitch fibers grow very little or not at all, according to most research investigation.

As the load imposed upon the muscles increases, the higher strata, faster twitch fibers—Type II ab and II b—must come into play or recruitment. Since these fibers (II ab and II b) are called upon when considerable force or tension is required, they are more adaptable to the growth or hypertrophy mechanism. How else would the body be able to meet increasingly more demanding loads if this adaptation was not available?

Have you ever noticed that in the general scheme of things most people can walk for considerable distances? They can normally jog for a lesser time and distance, and if you ask them to sprint, they won't go very far. The explanation for this pattern lies mainly in the recruitment of the different muscle fiber types necessary to perform at these progressively more demanding levels and their associated fueling systems. If a full-out sprint requires you to use your Type II b muscle fibers, you won't be able to sustain that high speed for long, because those muscle fibers don't have the endurance necessary—they are "fast twitch" and tire out quickly.

If we can adroitly manipulate the demand of the exercise routine, we can take advantage of the characteristics of loading, progression, and muscle system responses. There are obviously many different exercise plans, but almost NONE are actually based on an intricate awareness of these variables.

There are two major reasons for engaging in muscle "building" or growth. First, one of the primary supporters of actual muscle "growth" is the anabolic hormone system. The value of instigating increased muscle activity in the form of growth through high intensity training is that it significantly increases energy demand or calorie "burning." Obviously, using up stored body fat is one of our primary goals and, along with eating a controlled carb diet, muscle building exercise is a potent and indispensable component of any fat-reducing plan. So, when you perform an activity that calls upon every single muscle fiber, even Type II b, it stimulates growth, which then increases your metabolism and burns more calories. Second, the process stimulated by attempted muscle building, when successful, also generates increased bone mass, fat-burning hormone levels, energy levels, and cardiovascular and respiratory function. All of these changes contribute to increases in metabolic health and function and serve as youthful "anti-aging" mechanisms.

Muscle Fiber Recruitment: Low → High Intensity

Human beings have the capacity to move from a resting state to a high intensity situation instantaneously. This is related to our survival mechanism and running away from predators (or phone solicitors in today's world). The appropriate muscular reaction or recruitment can be initiated at the moment that the necessary stimulus or nerve impulse is transmitted, such as when you try to lift something heavy. The most intense, strenuous muscular forces or efforts can be sustained for short periods of time and lesser forces or efforts can continue longer. This entire sequence of events has everything to do with muscle action and fiber types and the energy systems that fuel or sustain them. The following diagram is meant to clarify and illustrate these concepts. Don't be discouraged if this chart seems a little technical, because most folks in the exercise field haven't mastered these concepts, in my opinion.

Muscle Fiber Chart

	Sugar	Fat			
Fibers	Glycolytic*	Oxidative*	Endurance*	Strength*	Energy pathway*
Type I	LOWEST	HIGHEST	HIGH	LOW	Aerobic
Type II a	↓	↑	↓	↓	Anaerobic/ Aerobic
Type II ab	↓	↑	↓	↓	Aerobic/ Anaerobic
Type II b	HIGHEST	LOWEST	LOW	HIGH	Anaerobic

In the above chart, "Glycolytic" simply describes the process during which these muscle fibers use "glycogen" (sugar) primarily. So, in lower intensity exercise, your Type I fibers are not using sugar to fuel their energy, but in higher intensity exercise when you call upon your Type II ab and Type II b, you are at the highest glycolytic state. "Oxidative" pertains to that condition wherein the working muscle fibers primarily use "the oxygen pathway," which must be combined with fat for fueling. When performing lower intensity, "steady state" cardio, your muscle fibers use the highest percentage of fat for fuel, while higher intensity resistance training uses less of a percentage of fat but just as much total fat in the fuel mixture. This later state is categorized as "glycolytic" or anaerobic—not relying primarily on the "oxygen" pathway.

"Endurance" refers to the following types of activities primarily associated with the recruitment or use of these muscle fibers: longer, slower, more prolonged activity. As discussed, Type I muscle fibers have the most endurance and are slow to tire out, whereas Type II b muscle fibers can only be used for short bursts of activity because they become exhausted much more quickly. On the flip side, "Strength" generally refers to the following types of activities primarily associated with the recruitment of these muscle fibers: shorter tem, more explosive, heavier types of exercises. Type I muscle fibers have the least strength, whereas Type II b fibers have the most strength.

"Energy Pathways" denotes which type of fuel—fat or sugar—is primarily used by these types of muscle fibers. (Caveat: In reality, all muscle fibers use some combination of fat and sugar, although the percentages can vary greatly.) Muscles can be fueled either aerobically or anaerobically, and it's usually some combination of the two. Aerobic fueling utilizes an oxidative or fat-burning system. This process is used during lower intensity activities that can be sustained for longer periods of time, such as walking. The muscle fibers that are generally recruited are the Type I and at a little higher demand, Type II a. In some rare instances, some Type II ab fibers might even be called upon.

Anaerobic fueling utilizes a glycolytic or sugar-burning system. This process is called upon at increasingly more demanding or intense levels of activity—for example, running very fast or exercising with highly demanding levels of resistance. This level of demand can only be sustained for shorter periods of time when Type II ab and Type II b fibers must be recruited. This process produces waste products or "exhaust" (to use a car analogy), which shuts it down. When there is a certain buildup of these waste products, fatigue occurs. The exerciser must slow down or decrease the weight, so that the lower strata Type I fibers, which can sustain their aerobic or longer lasting fueling, can continue handling the decreased load.

Whenever the higher Type II or faster twitch muscle fibers are working, the lower strata, slower twitch muscle fibers must be working as hard as they can, or the stronger fibers wouldn't be recruited or called upon. In simple terms, aerobic exercise *must* be encountered whenever anaerobic exercise is being sustained for some consequential duration. As a clarification, since muscle fiber types are called upon in a specific, consistent order, when some are working ALL of the lower strata fibers MUST be working as hard as they can or else they would NOT have to call upon and recruit the next higher level muscle fiber types. If we refer back to the muscle fiber chart, we can see that since the lower level fiber types (Type I or Type II a for example) have to be working first in order to demand the next higher fiber levels (Type II ab and Type II b), these lower level fibers (aerobic fibers) have to be fueled in their normal way (pathway), which is aerobically (primarily fat fueled). This means that when high intensity muscle work is being performed through high intensity (SMaRT) exercise BOTH aerobic and anaerobic fibers are working as hard as they can to try to respond to this high muscle demand.

It is certainly true that at higher levels of intensity, the aerobic, oxidative, or fat-burning fibers contribute to a lesser degree or percentage than they do at lower intensity, but they must be activated to their fullest capacity during high intensity exercise because the higher intensity glycolytic, sugar-burning fibers are being recruited. Therefore, this new contribution of glycogen or sugar to the fueling mixture reduces the percentage of the fat contribution, but you are still burning just as much overall fat. Remember, there will be more excess fat left in circulation after high intensity exercise, because the body "over shoots" fat release from storage because of the adrenaline surge. You should therefore NOT be "hungry" or forced to slow down metabolically, as in the aftereffect of long-term aerobic exercise.

For example, let's say we're doing a lower level, aerobic exercise that takes 10 units of energy per minute. Because the activity is not intense, the fuel mixture could be 8 calories per minute contributed by fat, with sugar/glycogen contributing the other 2 calories—a ratio of 80 percent fat burning per minute. Now, let's say we switch to a high intensity level of exercise that requires 30 calories per minute to fuel. In this case, 10 of the calories might be coming from fat while 20 might be coming from sugar/glycogen. We now have only a 33 percent contribution from fat. But while this is a smaller percentage of fat, it is still more total fat per unit of time (per minute).

Whenever you are exercising intensely, you are using fat and sugar. In fact, we are always using some combination of both fuels. The percentages change but the absolute values or levels of fat do not decrease during harder exercise. "Harder" exercise is simply that level of exercise that demands that the Type II ab and especially the Type II b muscle fibers have to be called upon to meet the high intensity demand. This can include wind sprinting (running), sprint swimming, high demand resistance training, or usually any activity that can only be sustained for 30 to 90 seconds at a time before local muscle failure occurs. This is an important concept, because it reveals that even during anaerobic exercise our bodies are still also in an aerobic mode and receiving those benefits. Now that we understand the science behind why anaerobic exercise recruits all of our muscle fibers for the maximum benefit, let's take a look at what I believe to be the best type of exercise for our bodies.

Traditional Resistance Training versus SMaRT Training

I use the term "resistance training" instead of weight lifting, strength training, and a number of other descriptives, because it includes all forms of resistance exercise from body weight, to dumbbells, to resistance bands, to Total Gyms, and so on. On Earth, all exercise is resistance training, since we live on a planet that provides a constant form of resistance force called gravity. A prudent, productive exercise plan takes advantage of the manipulation of simple, undeniable physical principles to our best advantage. This gives us the greatest "bang" for our exercise "buck." In this section, I will explain some of the basic terminology in the resistance training game, including reps, sets, muscle loading, load time, and mechanical failure.

"Reps" are repetitions, or the number of times a full exercise movement is performed. They normally consist of two parts: 1. Positive or concentric, moving the resistance from a starting (relaxed) position to a finished (contracted) position, and 2. Negative or eccentric, returning from contracted to start or relaxed position. Traditionally, people often perform around 10 repetitions of a particular exercise.

"Sets" are simply one series of repetitions (for example: 10 "reps") of the same movement, from the beginning to the end of that particular movement series. Most resistance programs use multiple sets of 6 to 12 repetitions and sometimes multiple exercises for the same muscle group. In many cases conventional programs are constructed of multiple sets of multiple exercises for the same muscle/groups, sometimes consisting of a total of 60 to 90 total repetitions for one muscle group. For example, you may decide to work the triceps muscles in your arms, so you complete three sets of 10 reps on one machine at the gym (for a total of 30 reps), and then three sets of 10 reps on two other similar machines, for a total of 90 reps that work your triceps.

"Load time" is simply the duration from the beginning of muscle contraction (involvement) in a set to the end of that tension time. For example, if you were to perform four reps taking 10 seconds each, the total "load time" for the set would be 40 seconds.

SMaRT training consists of only one set for each muscle group, and usually between 3 to 6 repetitions for that one muscle. For example, if you are working your triceps, you would now only do one machine, one set, and fewer reps. So compared to conventional training, the SMaRT exercise routine can consist of as little as 5 percent to 10 percent of the actual mechanical work traditionally encountered. Instead of focusing on the number of repetitions or sets like most conventional exercise programs, we emphasize the load time, or the duration of the muscle tension application.

An important aspect of load time and why we focus on it is the physiological tenet that muscles will work at the highest intensity for only short periods of time. Of course, the load time or duration of an exercise set is significantly influenced by the resistance that is selected. If that resistance is considered too "light," the load time will become too long (usually more than 90 seconds of constant load). Conversely, if the load time is too short (usually less than 30 seconds of constant load), the resistance is probably too "heavy." Remember, you are now engaging all muscle fiber types, including Type II b. Since we have established that stimulating high intensity muscle fibers through exercise provides the best return in the form of positive results for exercisers then it makes sense to address that mechanism. In simple terms, muscle physiology dictates that our time under high intensity load will practically correspond to a 30 to 90 second tension time (per set).

In almost all cases when a set of exercise exceeds the 90 second limit, it indicates a couple of possibilities: The resistance is insufficient (too light) and/or the load is intermittent. This means that there are essentially "rest" periods during the movement (usually a significant difference between the resistance curve of the device used and the user's strength curve). In that case, the resistance provided does NOT maintain high intensity load or muscle fiber recruitment. When following the SMaRT training program, you want to slowly, steadily complete each movement without any rest between reps. One of the tenets that I designed into slow resistance training as part of the program is the constancy of muscle load. Once a set is initiated, the goal is to maintain a high degree of consistent tension or mechanical demand until that load produces a level of failure. The muscle simply "gets too tired" to continue. When this occurs, you know that you have engaged and productively taxed all the muscle fibers, including the very important Type II b fibers.

In effect, every set of a SMaRT training workout is a mini "stress test." Each exercising muscle is progressively stressed or worked until it reaches a point of failure to continue at that demand level. The upside of this concept is that there is really no failing this test. If the resistance and the style (form) are reasonably controlled then that point described as momentary muscle failure (mechanical) correlates strongly to a "threshold" level metabolic state. THAT is the "signal" we are looking for in exercise. Once that point is reached, we have done virtually all we can do to stimulate positive muscle metabolism and all the associated support chemistry involved in that process. This includes "healthy" cardiovascular, respiratory, hormonal, skeletal and neurological adaptations.

• • •

Now that you understand the difference between exercise and activity, why cardio alone doesn't work, and the science behind why a high intensity resistance training program paired with a controlled carbohydrate diet results in the most optimal fat burning, you're ready for the five-week metabolic makeover, using the SMaRT program. You will learn how to properly exercise all of the major muscle groups to failure so that you engage all of the muscle fiber types, including the Type II b fibers, the holy grail of fat and sugar burning.

Most folks are surprised to discover how quickly they can *sense* a feeling of increased strength and energy and how they can actually *see* body changes after even two or three workouts. Your new way of eating will give you a sense of control and you will quickly appreciate that hunger is no longer a constant driver of your behavior. I bet you will be surprised by just how little it takes to obtain a maximum response. Now, let's get SMaRT!

PART II

The SMaRT™ Program

CHAPTER FOUR

THE FIVE-WEEK METABOLIC MAKEOVER

Most people who engage in an exercise and diet plan want to *change* something. It might be body fat, muscle tone, strength, health profile, cosmetic appearance, or performance capacity. In each case, the underlying driving force is changing your metabolism. I know many people believe that they are born with a certain metabolism; some feel "cursed" by theirs, but all is certainly not lost. If you don't think you can change metabolism, consider these events: puberty, pregnancy, holiday seasons, divorce, death, menstrual periods, and on and on. When these situations occur, something in your chemistry changes, and the result can be manifested in significant fluctuations in weight, body composition, mood, and a host of other alterations.

If you learn one thing from this book it should be that we induce change by sending different signals than those to which our bodies have become accustomed. Also remember that the signals have to be powerful enough and applied consistently enough to force the body to change its comfort zone or homeostasis. Now, what are the two most potent signal-changing behaviors? That's right—in most cases, diet and exercise. What kind of diet and exercise? That's correct, a controlled-carb diet and high intensity exercise. I told you exercise was good for the brain!

So what is it specifically that we are trying to accomplish? In the majority of cases, we are trying to produce higher levels of fat burning and muscle building. It is really that simple. The manipulation of the associated pathways (fat burning and muscle building) is the driving force for changing metabolism.

Low (controlled)-carb eating allows us to more readily "unlock" stored fat and reduce blood sugar fluctuations associated with problematic bouts of hunger, cravings, and sluggishness. High intensity exercise drives an adrenaline response that propels the release of fatty acids from storage that, in turn, increases available energy (making us more physically active) and provides fuel for better muscle tissue and bone tissue growth. That resulting lean tissue increase translates into a higher rate of resting and exercising levels of metabolic activity—your metabolism speeds up and you burn more calories. You become a fat burner instead of a fat storer. As an exaggerated example, I use the case of a crack addict. Did you ever see one of these poor folks? Because of the signals that this powerful chemical sends, these people are constantly moving and never hungry. They have *really* changed their metabolisms, but I wouldn't recommend that method!

Why the SMaRT Plan Works
(Hint: It's Metabolic)

The fact that the SMaRT system produces significant responses through the application of two 15-minute exercise sessions per week and a controlled carb diet raises some eyebrows—and it *should.* It sounds similar to many other claims conveniently made by sham programs. However, this book describes the differences in the application of the SMaRT exercises from those conventionally offered. This makes all the difference in the world with regard to legitimate metabolic changes in the form of reduced body fat and muscle gain.

Almost no programs achieve the muscle fiber recruitment and associated chemistry capable of producing the muscle building/fat burning metabolic pathways that the SMaRT system does. If this muscle fiber recruitment pattern that we discussed in chapter three is not addressed as the basis of any exercise program claiming substantial responses, you should be wary. This mechanism is, in fact, at the very heart of the metabolic matter.

Here's a long-term belief from years of consistent observation and repetition: Lean body mass—muscle and bone—is a vital and critical component in the formulation of increased metabolic rate. Only high intensity muscle demand can increase lean tissue in most adults. No amount of lower level exercise can substitute for a small amount of directly applied high intensity exercise for increased calorie burn. On the simplest level, we have to work muscles harder than they're used to in order to drive positive lean muscle tissue activity.

Many programs profess to be aware of this connection; however, almost none present reasonable, rational, safe applications of this concept. Instead, they claim their workout is killer, ultimate, blasting, and so on. But that's quite frankly just silly hype. Believe me, digging a twenty foot trench, six feet deep, with a pick and a shovel is killer, ultimate, and blasting, but it's *not* productive exercise! It will make you sore, tired, and enormously sweaty, but it will not increase fat burning in the long run.

The universal mountain in the fitness and health field is the burning or reduction of stored body fat. We've discussed the futility of this process throughout the last 50 years. Research, plans, systems, and programs have professed to provide successful vehicles for this process, but overwhelming evidence demonstrates the abject failure of this elusive objective. It's not working. Why? My observation is that a flawed concept of physiology has been consistently applied when addressing this dilemma. Simple caloric restriction doesn't work until a person reaches a state of semi-starvation, which is behaviorally an almost impossible long-term strategy. Burning calories through excessive, random, fuel-burning physical activities doesn't work either. The combination of the two produces fatigue, stress hormone escalation, and a metabolic slow down that ensures futility, behavioral irritability, and ultimate failure. So what's the alternative?

In my opinion, you can't beat this problem with a stick. You need an expertly applied behavioral scalpel. That tool requires a cutting edge application of dietary physiology and a mechanical intervention (exercise) that synergistically coordinates a metabolic makeover. It provides a powerful, logical strategy that defies tradition and opens a whole new realm of opportunity for long-term success.

A fairly large body of data exists that reinforces the possibility of losing a pound or two of weight a week, using a number of weight-loss methods. These methods are often a bit misleading, because most caloric restriction diets generate an equal muscle loss combined with fat loss. The net fat loss is one pound per week, which may sound fine, but the danger is that it also includes one pound of muscle loss, which means that your metabolic rate will decrease. Slowing down the speed at which you burn calories is not a formula for continued fat loss.

I believe that any program intended to positively change the metabolic milieu must include two pertinent issues: the composition of the diet and the chemistry induced by the exercise undertaken. Unless these two behaviors are addressed based upon some sound knowledge, expectations can range wildly. You shouldn't expect a nutritional plan that doesn't positively affect the way the body stores or burns fat to produce substantial results. By the same token, it would be futile to believe that an exercise regimen that borrows fat during its process and simply pays it back later into its reserve would be successful. Yet this is *exactly* what most diet/ exercise programs provide—little hope and low expectations.

On the other hand, if you were to apply an eating plan that is constructed to reduce the chemistry of fat storage and encourages the exaggerated utilization of fat as a primary fuel source, it would be reasonable to expect consistent reduction of stored body fat. With regard to appropriate exercise, a system that provokes the release of stored body fat would be preferred. In addition, it is incumbent upon a fat-loss system to drive increased muscle metabolism by instigating increased muscle mass. This two-pronged benefit provides the body with ample energy to sustain the demands of the applied exercise and have some energy leftover to combat fatigue and hunger and additionally keep calories burning at a higher metabolic rate 24/7.

If you apply a traditional weight-loss plan—low fat, low calorie, aerobic exercise—you can expect a pound or two of weight loss for the first few weeks. You may also experience low energy levels and common bouts of hunger. The long-term success rate is poor. However, the outcome and expectation levels for five weeks on the SMaRT system are as follows: a ten-pound reduction in body fat and an eight-pound increase in muscle tissue. This second element is significant because it provides a much better chance of long-term success. Behaviorally, much less hunger is reported and greater energy levels are consistently sustained. The chances for adherence to the program are vastly improved and the selection between the programs comes down to this: SMaRT or stupid!

My client Paul is a terrific example of why the five-week metabolic makeover program works so well. Paul was a 45-year-old, ex-high level football player. I've known Paul for about 30 years, and I call him "Big Pauli" for the simple reason that he is 6 feet 6 inches tall and weighs well over 300 pounds! He is a really BIG guy, but not a fat guy at all when in shape. Unfortunately, Paul had been busy establishing a highly successful business and fell off the fitness wagon.

He came to me saying that he wanted to really "hit it" and get back into top shape. I put Paul on the Five Week Metabolic Makeover Program. I had him cut out the wine and beer and drop the sugar and carbs dramatically, and we did ten 15-minute workouts (in 5 weeks) using the SMaRT protocol. Paul attacked the plan with the vengeance of the competitive athlete that still remained inside of him.

Paul's results were the most extreme I've ever witnessed! Caveat: Paul is NOT a typical human being. He was, at one time, lean and muscular at about 275 pounds! His results are more dramatic than any normal-sized person could attain but are an impressive example of what can be accomplished in a short period of time with minimal time allotted to the right kind of exercise.

Paul's results: In five weeks (a total of ten 15-minute workouts) Paul lost 50 pounds of fat and gained 35 pounds of muscle! His body literally undertook a metamorphosis! He seemed to visibly change every day I saw him. I use him in seminars to dramatically demonstrate the power of eating and exercising SMaRT!

Why Five Weeks?

A big part of designing a metabolic makeover is planning for success. I like to think that I stack the deck in every way possible, to the best of my ability, knowledge, and experience. Would I be so delusional as to attribute each facet of the plan some predetermined percentage toward a successful outcome? No . . . but why not use all the tools at our disposal? Understanding that humans are a fickle and fragile group, it has occurred to me that a short-term strategy is more palatable than a lifelong commitment, especially during the initiation phase of any behavioral change plan.

I have received very little pushback on a five-week "buy-in" to this idea. Most people can focus and remain disciplined for five weeks if the following occurs:

- They see some significant responses.

- They can comfortably incorporate the plan into a rational lifestyle.

- They get some honest, positive feedback.

That's exactly what we're about to do.

What can you expect? In a comprehensive study conducted in 2006, the *average* results from the Five-Week Metabolic Makeover Program included:

- A 10-pound fat loss

- An increase of 8 pounds of lean tissue

- A 30 percent decrease in body composition fat content

- A decrease in resting blood pressure and heart rate

- Upper and lower body strength gains of more than 25 percent

- An increase in trunk flexibility

These responses are normally enough to keep the trainee motivated to continue past the five weeks and incorporate the plan into a more permanent lifestyle regimen. Remember, these are the *average* results that I've witnessed during the last 40 years of training people with the my program. This means that some people achieved a quarter of these results while others had four times the average. Variables that should be taken into consideration include: starting condition or weight, age, gender, previously attained levels of leanness, hormonal status, support systems, and adherence levels. Still, for average results, these are phenomenal. A 10-pound loss in body fat is 10 times the result from conventional aerobic exercise!

Start with a Body Fat Analysis

What's more important: body weight, Body Mass Index (BMI), or body composition? It's important to understand the difference. Body weight simply indicates your mass, including tissues, fat, bone, muscle, and so on, regardless of your composition. It is a vague and potentially misleading indicator. Body Mass Index, commonly referred to as your BMI, is still a gross estimate of body tissue distribution. For example, most NFL running backs and linebackers, who are in great shape and have huge muscles, would be categorized as obese or morbidly obese by BMI standards. Body composition, measured by a number of reasonable methods, is a much more relevant indicator of the state of your fitness and health status.

And, in my experience, no one really cares what they weigh. I know you find that hard to believe, and maybe you care about that number on the scale. But if I told you that you could weigh 10 more pounds but look like Heidi Klum, I'm sure you'd be fine with that! Many people would love to be 12 percent body fat or less, despite the actual body weight involved. Most people want to use exercise and diet to improve their body composition—how much of their bodies are comprised of muscle and how much are composed of fat. Leanness does not equal skinniness. It is the presence of muscle and the absence of fat, and that's the real universal goal—metabolically and aesthetically.

So the most sensible place to start a metabolic makeover is with a simple assessment of your metabolic status by obtaining a body composition. A body fat analysis is simply a test that measures and breaks down weight into lean mass and fat mass. There are a number of reasonably reliable methods. A DEXA scan is the most accurate but expensive and, for our purposes, an unnecessary luxury. If you have access to underwater measurement (hydrostatic method), electronic impedance, Bod Pod, and some infrared techniques, they will all do. There is, of course, debate as to the accuracy of each, but they all seem to indicate whether you are losing or gaining fat and/or lean tissue, and that is the real purpose of the measurement. Many moderate to high level exercise facilities have some resource or mechanism for determining one's body composition; if not, we will provide a method you can use at home.

An important reminder: The scale can be a very inaccurate tool when measuring metabolic progress—especially regarding the all-important fat-loss factor. Remember, in the famous SMaRT study, the average result was a 10-pound fat loss but an 8-pound lean tissue (muscle and bone) gain. That's only a 2-pound change on the scale BUT waistlines and hips reduced significantly in size (pants and skirt sizes), and the appearance of muscle "shape" was visibly more pronounced. Muscle is denser than fat and therefore is a lot heavier. Lean weight is almost never a problem with regard to metabolic or cosmetic considerations. Body composition is the key to health and cosmetic measurement not simple body weight.

Women

Step 1: Measure your body weight using a weight scale and record the result; for example, 140 pounds.

Step 2: Wrap a cloth tape measure around your wrist at its thickest point and record the girth; for example, 7 inches.

Step 3: Wrap the tape measure around your waist, level with your navel, and record the result; for example, 28 inches.

Step 4: Measure around your hips at the widest point and record the result; for example, 39 inches.

Step 5: Measure around your forearm at the fullest point and record that number; for example, 10 inches.

Step 6: Enter your measurements in the following formula to calculate fat mass:

Fat Mass = Weight –[(Weight x 0.732) + 8.987 + (Wrist / 3.14) + (Waist x 0.157) + (Hip x 0.249) + (Forearm × 0.434)]

In the example, the formula would break down as follows:

Fat Mass = 140 – [(140 x 0.732) + 8.987 + (7 / 3.14) – (28 x 0.157) – (39 x 0.249) + (10 x 0.434)]

Fat Mass = 140 – [102.48 + 8.99 + 2.23 - 4.4 – 9.71 + 4.34]

Fat Mass = 140 – 103.93

Fat Mass = 36.07

Step 7: Divide your fat mass by your body weight and multiply by 100 to calculate percent body fat. In the example, 36.07 divided by 140 times 100 calculates a percent body fat of 25.76 percent.

Men

Step 1: Weigh yourself on a weight scale and record the result; for example, 220 pounds.

Step 2: Wrap a tape measure around your waist and record the amount; for example, 44 inches.

Step 3: Enter the results in the following formula to calculate fat mass:

Fat Mass = Weight – [(Weight × 1.082) + 94.42 – (Waist × 4.15)]

In the example, this formula calculates fat mass as follows:

Fat Mass = 220 – [238.04 + 94.42 – 182.6]

Fat Mass = 220 - 149.86

Fat Mass = 70.14

Step 4: Divide your fat mass by your body weight. Multiply by 100 to calculate percent body fat. In the example, 70.14 divided by 220 times 100 calculates a percent body fat of 31.88 percent.

Lab Work

Additionally, if you have the coverage and /or the money to order labs (actually have your doctor order them), you can have a blood draw to include measurements of triglycerides, blood glucose, A-1C hemoglobin, HDL/LDL cholesterol levels, C-reactive protein, and/ or homocysteine. These are all relevant indicators of metabolic health:

- Triglycerides: Remember, these are the packages of fat that are stored and circulate in our bodies to provide fat for fuel. An overload of triglyceride is associated with a myriad of health problems. Normal range of blood triglyceride = 140 – 200.

- Blood glucose: This is simply the measurement of sugar circulating in the blood that is tightly regulated for healthy brain and organ function. Normal range (fasting) = below 100.

- A-1C Hemoglobin: This measurement indicates how much blood sugar is present on a continued or long-term basis (not just at time of test like blood glucose). Hemoglobin is a protein that "turns over" approximately every 90 days, so this measurement is a great way to determine the blood sugar status on a longer term, more relevant basis. Healthy range = below 5.5.

- HDL/LDL cholesterol levels: This ratio of lipoproteins (the little "envelopes" that carry blood fats around) is a much more relevant indicator of health risk than a total cholesterol number. A good ratio for healthy risk level assessment = 3.5:1 or less (meaning that total cholesterol divided by HDLs should be in a ratio of 3.5 to 1 or less).

- C-Reactive protein and homocysteine: These inflammatory markers are used as indicators of levels of inflammation. C-Reactive protein is a marker of systemic inflammation—it doesn't tell us where the inflammation exists, just that it does. One gram per liter or less is considered low risk and as that number increases, so does corresponding inflammatory mediated health (usually heart) risk. In a homocysteine measurement,any reading above 15 mm/liter is considered to begin the high risk range for this amino acid that correlates to hardening of arteries and associated health risks.

It's informative to have some objective, baseline data when you start. Body composition is a great gross indicator and the blood work is a nice bonus feature!

After five weeks you should be able to retest and have some real, objective feedback on the level of success of your makeover. Most folks just *feel* much better—pants are looser, clothes fit better, and people ask you what you've been doing—but these tests just don't lie.

SMaRT Tips for Success

One of the uniquely advantageous elements of the SMaRT plan is the individually flexible format it provides. Some people have limited time, whether they are high-powered business executives or stay-at-home parents—and this program enables them to maximize their time. I have actually had many clients who literally ONLY did the two high intensity SMaRT sessions each week. It honestly impresses me that they attain and maintain high levels of health, body composition, and energy levels with this minimal lifestyle input—and it just shows how well this program works and why utilizing your muscles in this way has such global health benefits.

My experience has provided me with some observations for what appears to work best for people who want to obtain the most positive results. I've noticed that people who are "active" in addition to adhering to the twice weekly SMaRT sessions seem to achieve the most consistent long-term success. These activities are rec-ommended to those who choose to do them and certainly have no "downside" in the program unless they are overdone to the point of extreme fatigue. My advice is to choose other activities you enjoy that will fit into your schedule (we'll discuss exercise and activ-ity planning in the next chapter). I engage in stationary cycling, walking, and golf on my "off" days, because I like the activities and feel good doing them. The most common supplementary activi-ties include yoga, recreational sports like golf or tennis, and hiking. Make your own plan . . . and be SMaRT!

Some people find it helpful to log their workouts, diet, and prog-ress. There are so many online and computer programs available now to log your activity and eating. Find one if you like and use it to keep track of your exercise and activities. I still use an appointment book to log eating and activity each day. It gives me a real blueprint for assessing any fluctuations in weight, energy, body composition, and so on.

Although I am not a huge proponent of specific eating before or after high intensity exercise, I have observed and applied a few tips: Don't eat a big meal an hour or two before your workout, don't eat any carbohydrate (high energy) food after working out for a few hours (probably never on a low-carb diet), and a good protein snack or meal is fine an hour or so after a session. There is some evidence that the stimulation of HGH (human growth hormone) associated with high intensity exercise is enhanced by this after workout prac-tice. Again, it can't hurt.

Perhaps one of the most important elements for success is having a SMaRT plan mind-set. A lot of successful behavioral change involves determination and a dogged drive to do the best you can. The changing of metabolic status is not an easy undertak-ing. If it were simple, most people would be metabolically healthy. That would manifest itself in more fit and healthy people and a significantly diminished level of fat-related health disorders. I think of this corrective process as analogous to chopping down a big, old tree in your yard. One day you determine that that sucker is coming down, no matter what! Then every day you focus on doing what you can to make a dent in that thing. Some days, you wake up and it looks like it grew back again, but you stay focused and keep chopping.

Be cognizant of any of the variables involved, especially if you find yourself having difficulty. Are your carbs where you want them? Are you completing two good workouts per week? Are you getting solid sleep? If the answer to all of these questions is yes, then you might have to "tighten" up and make sure there are fewer latitudes and fluctuations. The more you engage in positive eating and exercise behaviors with consistency, the better your shot at success.

This is a program with a repeated, long-term track record of success. The majority of participants actually do achieve a high level of positive change. You can reasonably expect rapid and steadily enhanced levels of fat reduction, bio-markers for health, cosmetic benefits, and performance development, if you remain determined and follow the plan.

CHAPTER FIVE

THE SMART WORKOUT

Now we will begin the first part of the five-week metabolic make-over, which is the SMaRT Exercise program. This workout trains the whole body, from the largest muscles to the smallest muscles. The body doesn't grow an arm and a leg and a chest muscle separately; it grows as a unit. In the old days when someone came to me and said he was working hard but couldn't get his chest or arms to "grow," I would routinely ask him what exercise he did for his back and legs. I would then explain that his difficulty might stem from the body's resistance to disproportionate growth. In other words, working some selected muscle or group of muscles to the exclusion of other major muscle groups is usually a less than optimal plan. The exercises in the SMaRT workout will generate global and local responses throughout your body, sending the right signals to increase your metabolism and fat-burning. As noted in chapter three, there are so many benefits offered by exercise that a change in diet alone can't offer. The best news? Even if you do not follow the controlled carbohydrate plan that I recommend in chapter six, you will still see significant changes in your body from the workout alone.

There are a number of myths about exercise, and people repeatedly ask me the same questions, such as "How often should I change my exercise routine?" If the exercise routine addresses strength, endurance, and flexibility adequately and consistently like the SMaRT program, it may never need to be changed. I've been doing this routine for more than 40 years! The reason I haven't changed my exercise regimen is that I still have the same muscles that perform the same functions that I had 40 years ago. My routine consistently challenges my major muscle groups within their major functions and instigates significant global support every time I perform that routine. There is no such thing as "muscle confusion"—it's simply a manufactured rationale for sending people multiple DVDs to fill a commercial package. Muscles never get used to working to failure by its very definition.

I have also been asked countless times over the years by over-enthusiastic, younger male trainees to "really beat them up and make them sore." I usually ask them to come into my back office where I keep a baseball bat, and I assure them that I can make them very sore, very quickly, but it probably won't do them much good! It is not uncommon for a new activity to produce significant soreness. One of the more common ways to induce soreness, for example, is to play in the company softball game once a year. Most of us agree that recreational, picnic softball is not the most demanding or effective way to exercise, but I can assure you that there are huge numbers of sore folks the next day as a result. Well-planned exercise, at any level of intensity, should produce little soreness and certainly not on a regular basis. Soreness is not indicative of a good workout. Muscle soreness has much more to do with disturbing the attaching system (tendons) than it does with exercising intensely or productively.

I've included three different SMaRT exercise programs that you can follow every week: One program can be followed by using the equipment at your local gym. There's a second program that can be followed at home using resistance bands. Lastly, for those of you who own or have access to a Total Gym machine, I've presented the SMaRT Total Gym workout. The SMaRT workout routines are plans that are truly flexible and can promote a high degree of success for anyone. Choose whichever of the three program plans works best for your lifestyle and, remember, you only *have* to exercise 30 minutes per week!

The Basic SMaRT Resistance Exercises for Your Metabolic Makeover

The foundation of your metabolic makeover exercise program are the twice per week resistance exercise sessions. There should be at least two days between each session, so a Monday/Thursday, Tuesday/Friday, Wednesday/Saturday type of schedule works best. These are the only mandatory, formal exercise sessions! Each one is only 15 minutes, so that's a total of 30 minutes of *required* exercise per week. That said, as mentioned in chapter three, it's always good to remain active in order to counteract sedentary behavior. The chart below provides some ideas for incorporating other activities into your schedule, as time allows.

While the SMaRT workouts are the only mandatory exercises in the above chart, you will see that I've added "advised," "suggested," and "optional" workouts as well. Years of observation and practice have taught me that being "active" is helpful and healthy. Advised workouts may include cardio activities, such as walking, hiking, biking, or tennis. If you don't have the time or inclination, don't become discouraged. If your eating is disciplined, you may need only to avoid sedentary behavior (sitting for hours at a time). Please don't fall into the traditional mindset that doing "more" will burn more calories, creating an energy (calorie) deficit. That is NOT our goal. Our exercise requirement is completely satisfied by our two SMaRT sessions. Activity doesn't hurt, but the calories "burned" are very much an overrated, futile, and vastly irrelevant concept in our metabolism altering program!

Here is the main consideration: The activity (or if you prefer, "other" exercise) that you incorporate along with the SMaRT workout twice a week routine, must NOT be so intense or deeply demanding that it interferes with the very important "recovery" phase (two days "off") of the process. Many folks chose to run a few miles on some off days. It has not seemed to interfere with recovery in my experience, but they don't do wind sprints or run distance to a point of near failure. That severe level of muscular demand can and will prove to be nonproductive and usually counterproductive in the long run (pun intended).

The SMaRT Chart of Dr. Ben's Weekly Workout Schedule

The 15-minute SMaRT Resistance Exercises must be performed twice a week. You can add to these mandatory exercises an advised or suggested activity and optional recreational activities.

	Sunday	Monday	Tuesday	Wednesday	Thursday	Friday	Saturday
Mandatory 15-Minute SMaRT Resistance Exercises		SMaRT™			SMaRT™		
You Can Add Advised Option	Cardio or Activity		Cardio or Activity			Cardio or Activity	
You Can Add Suggested Option	Flex	Flex	Flex	Flex	Flex	Flex	Flex
Optional Activities	Recreation			Recreation			Recreation

Suggested workouts, which you will notice are every single day, have to do with maintaining flexibility. I *strongly* suggest this because as we get older, we often lose mobility due to a loss of flexibility. I think that some stretching each day is an effort that produces wonderful returns. This can include yoga, Pilates, or even some simple stretches. I've outlined a basic stretching plan below that includes some simple, helpful stretches.

The optional "normal activities" category incorporates recreational activities like golf, horseback riding, or going on a nature walk with a friend. They do get your body moving, but since they tend to be hobbies we enjoy, we don't view them as traditional exercise or as a chore. I have found that people who enjoy leisure recreation and physical activities have a better, more healthful attitude about life and that the resulting positive chemistry is strongly related to good health and vitality. But if some of these choices become overwhelmingly obligatory and stressful, they might very well cause as much of a negative effect as the positive attributes they can produce, so think of them as enjoyable optional activities rather than something you absolutely MUST do every couple of days.

Can I Do the SMaRT Program If I'm Pregnant?

Women often wonder if it's safe to follow the program when they are pregnant. I have never had a problem with SMaRT training during pregnancy with my clients, but I would always advise someone to first seek approval from her physician if she is pregnant and wants to start an exercise program. Everyone is different, and it's always best to be safe!

Dr. Ben's Basic Stretching Routine

As a suggested part of The SMaRT Lifestyle Plan, I recommend some stretching, especially as we get older, but we're never too young to start. You can stretch every day, even on SMaRT Exercise days. Stretching does not interfere with any form of optional, suggested, or mandatory exercise or activity. If one chooses to stretch, this is a good, basic routine.

I personally stretch for 5–7 minutes every morning and every night. I have lost some flexibility as most folks do when they approach 70 years of age, but I find it relaxing and helpful in maintaining my range of motion for my golf game and in performing everyday tasks, such as getting in and out of my car.

There are many good flexibility programs available, and yoga is a great way for many people to fit in a suitable stretching session. The following are some of my favorite, simple stretches for the major problematic areas. Please don't feel restricted to these, but find those that work for you and be consistent with their performance.

I like to do many stretches lying on the floor as opposed to leaning over, for example. It's more stable and imposes much less stress on the spine. I also use a rolled up, good-sized towel under my neck when I'm lying on my back to reduce stress on the cervical spine (neck). I recommend holding the stretches in a position wherein tension, not pain or strain, is felt and then trying to relax in a stretched position for 10–20 seconds with very little "bouncing" involved. I have found repeating each stretch 2–4 times is sufficient for me. Try to adjust the variables to your liking.

SITTING HAMSTRING STRETCH

Sit on the floor—on a carpet or mat. I like my back supported by something, such as the bed or wall. Keep feet directly in front of you with knees reasonably straight. Slowly work both hands down the legs, from the thighs to the knees to the shins, and finally your feet, to a point of muscle tension or slight resistance. You should feel a stretching sensation in the lower back, hips, and hamstrings, even the back of your calves. Hold the stretch for 10 to 20 seconds, and try to relax to the point where you might increase the range of motion.

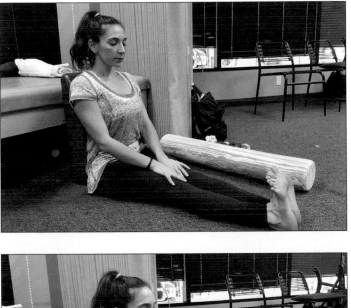

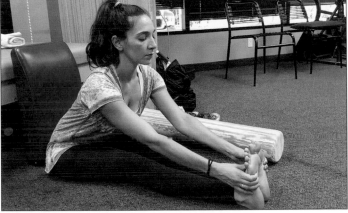

SITTING WIDE LEG BACK, HAMSTRING, AND HIP STRETCH

From the same sitting position as stretch number 1, spread your legs out as wide as comfortable. You can stretch forward, with your hands toward the middle, or you can stretch your left arm toward your right foot and right arm toward your left foot. Again, hold stretched positions for 10 to 20 seconds and repeat.

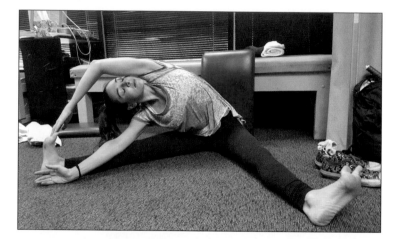

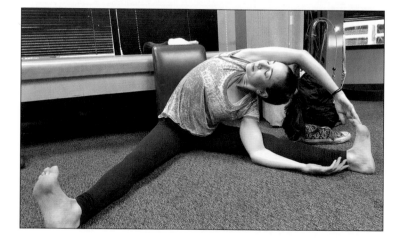

BENT KNEE SITTING GROIN STRETCH

Sit with your heels touching and your knees bent out toward your sides. Apply light tension to the inside of the thighs to feel a stretch on the inside of your thighs and relax. Hold for 10 to 20 seconds and repeat.

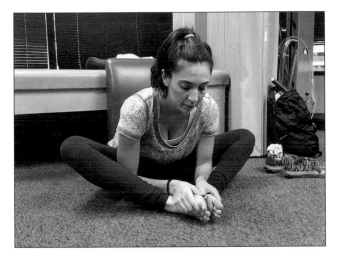

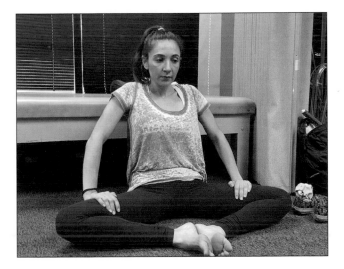

LYING TOWEL HAMSTRING STRETCH

Place a towel under your neck for support. Lie on your back and wrap a large towel around one foot. Pull straight leg back toward your head and hold at the point of tension, trying to relax the butt, hamstring, and back of calf. Switch legs and again hold for 10 to 20 seconds, trying to relax and stretch a little farther.

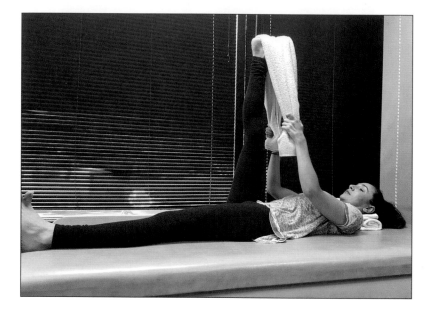

LYING ROTATIONAL HIP STRETCH

Lie on your back with a towel under your neck and knees bent at 90 degrees. Simply roll your legs (together) from one side to the other and hold each for 10 seconds. This stretch is great for loosening up the lower back.

LYING GLUTE STRETCH

Lie on your back with a towel under your neck. With your hands clasped around one knee, pull that knee back and hold stretch. Switch legs and repeat, holding stretch 10 to 20 seconds. This simple, basic stretch is good for your hips and lower back.

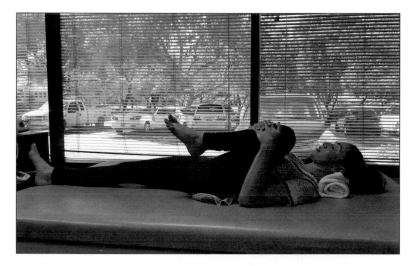

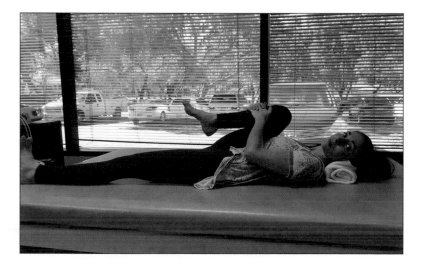

LYING SCIATIC NERVE HIP STRETCH

Lying on the floor, with a towel under your neck, bend your knees as in the former stretch. Pull one knee back and across the opposite leg. Hold the right knee with the right hand and pull back and across. With the left hand, pull your ankle back and across so that you can feel your femur (upper leg bone) rotating right in the middle of the glute (butt). This is where the problematic sciatic nerve leaves the hip area into the leg where it causes so much pain so often. Simply switch legs and arms and repeat.

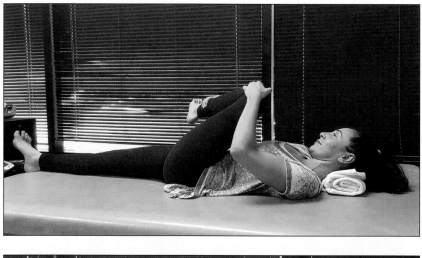

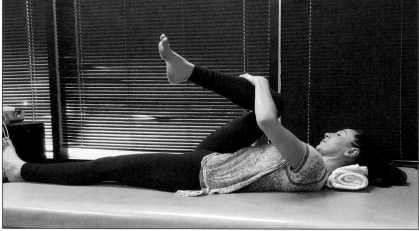

EAR TO SHOULDER TRAP STRETCH

Traps, the muscles that run from the back of the skull to the back of the shoulder and upper back, are the most commonly tight or in a state of spasm in most people. This causes neck discomfort and pain, and restricted movement. In a standing position, simply hold the right arm hanging at your side with the left arm at the elbow. Now let the head tilt away so that the left ear stretches toward the left shoulder and hold. Now reverse the stretch and hold the left arm with the right arm at the elbow. This stretch provides immediate and significant relief for most "stiff neck" sufferers.

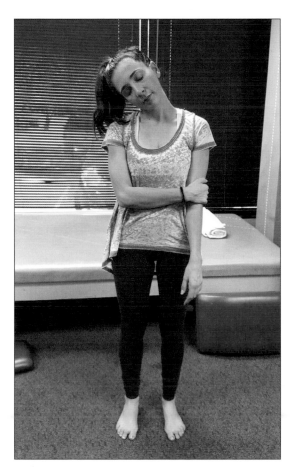

Some Simple SMaRT Guidelines
for all Exercise Routines

Before we delve into the exercise instructions for each of the three SMaRT workout programs, there are a few basic guidelines that apply to all three exercise routines. These general instructions have proven to support high levels of success by those engaging in SMaRT training:

1. Work large muscles first and proceed in a general sequence to smaller muscles/groups.

For example, proceed from hips and legs to torso (lats), shoulders, chest, arms, and so on (as shown in photo sequences). More effort is exerted with these large muscles, and they "set up" the enormous cardiovascular benefit of the routine most effectively.

2. Perform one set of each exercise to a point of mechanical failure.

That "failure"—or inability to complete a full repetition in good, controlled form—should be accomplished in a time frame of between 30 to 90 seconds of load time in almost every case. "Load time" is simply the elapsed time from the start of the set to the end. Most mobile phones have great stop watch apps—use them.

General rule of thumb: If you cannot achieve 30 seconds, the resistance or weight is probably too heavy. If you can easily reach the 90-second mark—and may even feel you can continue longer—the weight is probably too light. Make the adjustment in the next session. The first time you do an exercise, start with a resistance that feels "light" to simply get a sense of how to properly perform the exercise. You can increase resistance immediately if it feels like it is not a challenge and then use that as your starting point going forward.

Remember, the resistance you select for each exercise will ultimately depend on how long it takes you to perform slow repetitions until failure is reached. The weight or resistance will also likely be different for each exercise.

3. Rest between sets (exercises) as little as necessary to regain a controlled rate of breathing.

Move on to the next exercise when your breathing is not overly taxing. In other words, you should not be gasping or seriously laboring for breath before engaging in the next exercise. It's okay to be breathing at a higher than normal rate, just not to the extent that it will compromise your effort in the next set. However, this is NOT meant to suggest that there is a *rest*. I'd rather call it a *pause*. This recovery time should actually decrease in duration as you become more globally fit. At some point, some people can actually complete the entire routine with only the pause to get to the next machine or exercise before reengaging.

Breathing should NOT be regulated by count or position. It is natural for the body to respond by breathing heavily when performing high intensity exercise. Let it happen. This demonstrates the "global" or aerobic benefits driven by this form of exercise.

4. In most cases the entire routine can be encapsulated into 6–10 exercises.

The specific number of exercises will depend on equipment availability and any anatomical considerations or adaptations that might arise. I have provided specific instructions for 7 commercial gym exercises, 7 at-home rubber cable exercises, and 7 Total Gym™ exercises.

5. The speed of movement should be as slow and steady as feasible and the tension applied consistently throughout the entire range of motion.

This includes both during the positive (lifting) phase and the negative (returning) phase. The change in direction should be smooth, reducing bouncing or rebounding as much as possible. Always strive to move very slowly, maintaining tension or "load" on the exercising muscles both up and down on each exercise. Focus and visualize each movement in order to take advantage of the brain-muscle neurological connection.

6. Take at least two days off for the next SMaRT session.

Twice a week is the optimal sequencing of the SMaRT protocol to allow for adequate recovery and adaptation (results). MORE is NOT Better! If you really want to be exercising more than twice a week, refer to The SMaRT Chart for suggested complementary activities to safely supplement your program.

SMaRT Workout Tips

- Maintain proper form and posture.
- Breathe naturally.
- Move quickly between exercises.
- Do the SMaRT routine twice a week.
- Rest for two days between workouts.
- Stay focused/concentrate.
- Be consistent.

My Own Experiences—Three Ways

I have had personal success using each of the three following routines at some point, while performing the SMaRT exercise system on various kinds of commercial equipment, a Total Gym machine, and with resistance bands. The system simply works because the fundamental principles are sound and productive using most forms of resistance.

The foundation of the SMaRT system is universally applicable, regardless of equipment availability. If the tenets of slow movement carried to a point of muscle failure in a given time framework of 30 to 90 seconds, twice a week are adhered to, then good things begin to happen and continue to do so for a lifetime. That's just SMaRT!

The Commercial Gym
SMaRT Workout

For those of you who belong to a traditional gym, I've created a program based around the machines that most gyms offer. Since you will be working your muscles in a specific order—large to small—it's best if you complete these exercises in the order they are presented. It's important to follow proper form as you perform each exercise, so if you are uncertain about any of the instructions, review the accompanying photographs. This workout includes eight exercises that work the muscles in your legs, back, shoulders, chest, and arms. Be sure to complete all of them unless there is some unusual pain or discomfort experienced. These movements should NOT hurt, other than some fatigue-related discomfort, sometimes called a "burn."

LEG EXTENSIONS

Leg extensions work the quadriceps or what we often refer to as "quads." These are the four major muscles located on the front of the thighs. This exercise moves or extends the lower leg out in a kicking-type of motion.

Sit with the back support touching your lower back, with your knees set just in front of the seat pad and straight out from the hips. Slowly extend and straighten your lower legs against the foot pad situated at the bottom of your legs, just above ankle level. Extend them as high as possible without any kicking or jerking of the weight. Hold for about one second in this top position, creating as much tension as possible, even if movement stops. Return the weight slowly back to the starting bent leg position, resisting the weight continuously rather than "letting" the weight down. Touch the bottom position and immediately and subtly start the next repetition. Continue until you cannot perform a full repetition in good, controlled form. That "failure" should occur within a 30 to 90 second time frame.

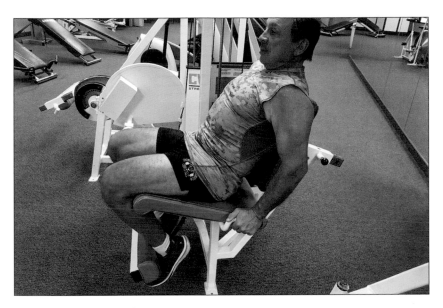

LEG EXTENSIONS – Start

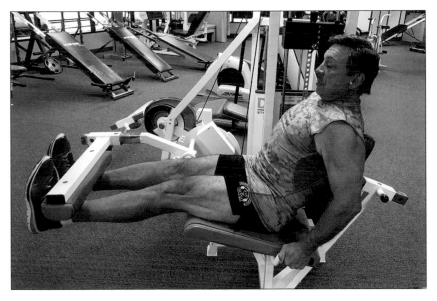

LEG EXTENSIONS – Finish

LEG CURLS

This exercise works the hamstrings—the three muscles on the back side of the upper legs, opposite the quadriceps above. These muscles bend the leg at the knee so that the heel draws back in an arc toward the butt. In my experience, these are crucial muscles involved in maintaining hip and lower back function and stability. I have *never* seen a person with good range and good strength in his or her hamstrings who had a low back problem, and, reciprocally, I have never seen a person with low back problems who didn't have tight and/or weak hamstrings. Depending on equipment availability, the resistance for leg curls is generally lighter than leg extensions.

To start the exercise (usually lying prone, on abdomen), place your kneecaps just off the bench pad. Knees should be extended straight out with foot pad positioned just above ankle height on the back of the lower leg. Keeping butt down so that hips don't rise off the bench, slowly bend the knees to bring the feet up to the butt in an arc to at least 90 degrees, unless that position becomes unattainable due to tightness or extreme weakness at that position. Think of doing an arm curl for biceps, except use your legs to do so. Again, continue until you cannot attain that 90 degrees of bending. That failure should occur within 30 to 90 seconds. Don't be surprised if your hamstrings "fail" very abruptly. That is not uncommon.

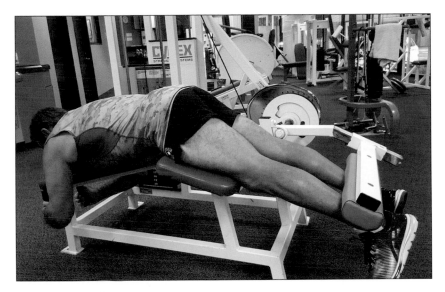

LEG CURLS – Start

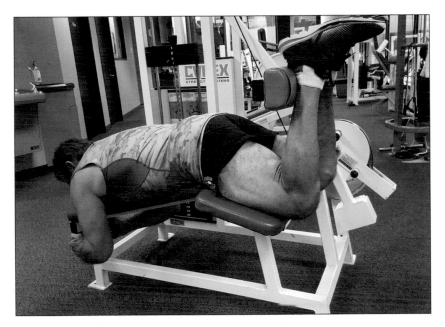

LEG CURLS – Finish

The "seated" version of the leg curl is performed by starting in a seated position (similar to the leg extension exercise), except this time the legs are extended straight out and the foot pad is positioned on the back of the lower leg, above the ankle. The move is a simple bending at the knee, drawing the heel back up toward the butt in an arc. Speed and fatigue principles follow the same directions as for every SMaRT exercise.

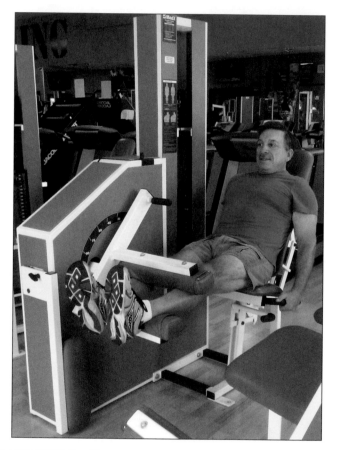

SEATED LEG CURLS – Start

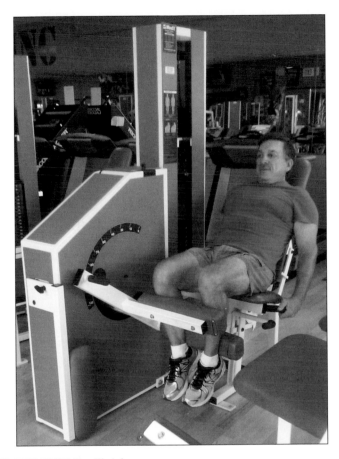

SEATED LEG CURLS – Finish

ROWING

This exercise works the largest muscles of the back/upper back, known as the lats and traps (latissimus and trapezius). These muscles cover the entirety of the back—from the back of the skull and shoulders all the way down to the lower third and side of the back of the body. These muscles primarily (but not exclusively) pull the shoulders down and back. They are incredibly powerful and multifunctional (do a lot of movements) muscles/groups.

Sit with the handles at about chest height or a little lower. Position your elbows slightly lower than shoulder height, out to the sides. The starting position should be one that stretches your shoulders forward to the point where you feel a stretch across the upper back. From that position, slowly pull the elbows back, feeling a pinching or retraction in the shoulder blades. It is helpful to think about pulling with the shoulder blades rather than the arms. This is strictly a kinesthetic "feel" idea but helpful to understand and isolate the intended upper back muscles.

Pull the elbows back past the body plane as far as possible without jerking the body backward. It is certainly allowable for the body to "lean" back slightly, so that the chest comes off the chest support. Folks who want the contact with the chest support to remain in full forward position are reducing the likelihood of full, large muscle exercise (as intended) and reducing the exercise to the limitation of the smaller rhomboid muscles (little muscles in the upper back). Again, failure occurs when the elbows can no longer pull back beyond the plane of the body in good, controlled form.

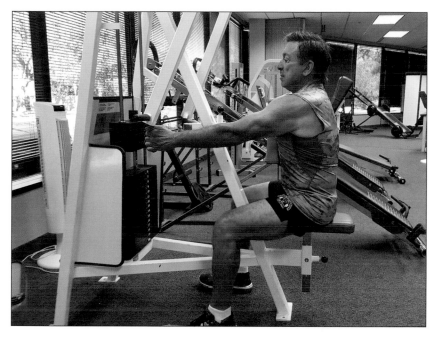

ROWING – Start

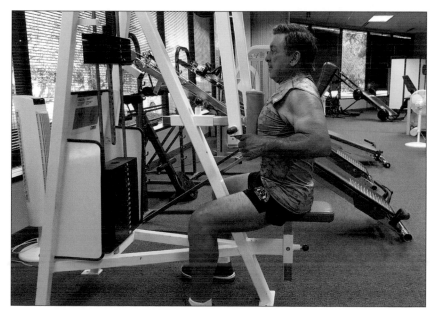

ROWING – Finish

LATERAL RAISES

This exercise works the shoulder muscles. Sit with your upper arms at your sides, elbows bent, and forearms straight. Grip the handles in front of you—forearm pads should be resting on top of your forearms. Slowly raise bent arms out to sides, with elbows leading the action, and return to your sides. Keep the upper arms on a plane even with the body (not in front or behind that plane). This exercise isolates the deltoid or shoulder muscles, which are largely composed of fast twitch, fast fatiguing fibers.

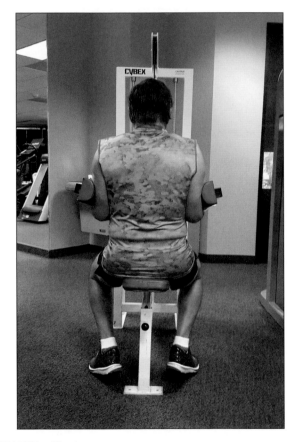

LATERAL RAISE – Start

The resistance will become "heavy" rapidly, so that very few repetitions can produce fatigue quickly. The load time for this exercise might well be 30 to 45 seconds. These muscles are usually easy to "feel" and isolate. When you can no longer raise your upper arms to approximately 90 degrees, you will be done with that set.

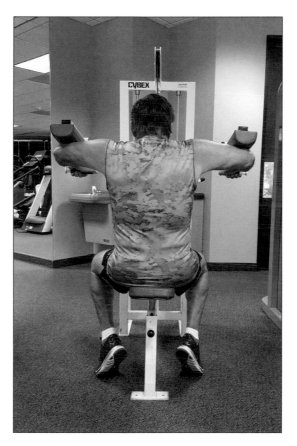

LATERAL RAISE – Finish

CHEST/PEC FLIES

This exercise works the chest muscles. Even though the chest muscles/pectorals are multi-functional—involved in a number of different shoulder girdle movements—this exercise provides a competent taxation of the entire complex.

Sit with your upper arms situated at approximately shoulder level out to the sides, with elbows bent and forearms raised upward, resting on arm pads. The ideal position would be with the upper arm in a slightly elevated angle upward, but many people have trouble and discomfort in this position, so I suggest finding a comfortable position. The start or stretched position should also be one that feels muscularly stretched but not strained at the joint in any way. From that position, apply tension to the arm pads at the elbow and forearm rather than a strong hand grip position. Feeling tension, move from the front of the shoulder to the sternum, slowly squeeze pads or handles to the front of the chest and return slowly concentrating on the chest rather than the shoulders or arms.

As in all exercises, repeat until an approximately full range position cannot be achieved. There will be a slightly decreased range of motion at the end of the movement, since the strength curve of most diverts considerably from the resistance curve of most machines, decreasing considerably near the finished position.

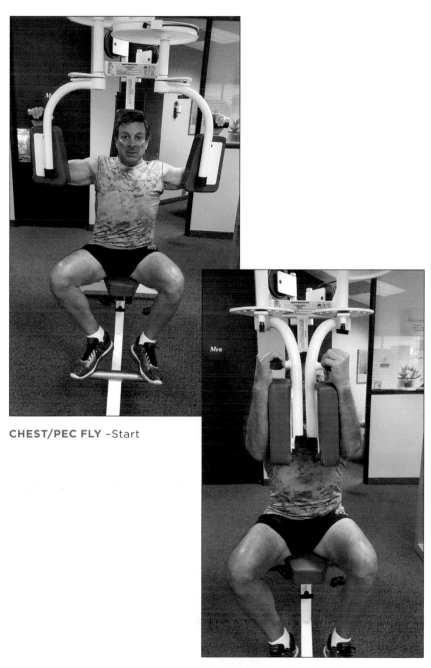

CHEST/PEC FLY –Start

CHEST/PEC FLY – Finish

SEATED DUMBBELL CURLS

This exercise works the biceps or "bending" muscles in front of the upper arm. Sit with your back supported and a dumbbell in each hand, with palms pointing straight forward and fully extended at your sides. Slowly bend both arms toward you in an arc that finishes with your hands in front of your shoulders and then slowly return to starting position. Remember, this exercise produces an "arc," not a straight line. Continue until you can no longer perform a full repetition in good form. If your back begins to arch and your body moves around for leverage, the set should be over.

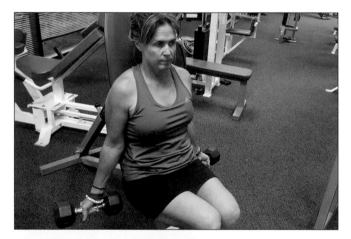

SEATED DUMBBELL CURLS – Start

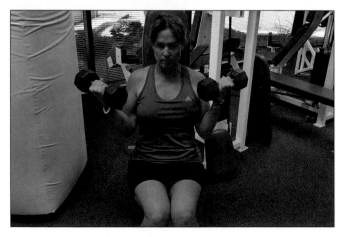

SEATED DUMBBELL CURLS – Finish

You can also do this exercise using the bicep curl machine at the gym, following similar movements. Sit with your arms straight out in front of you, elbows resting on the pad and palms up, gripping the bar in front of you. Slowly raise the bar toward you, until right in front of your face. Slowly return to starting position.

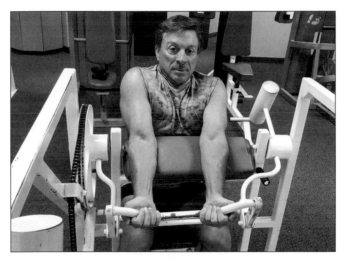

MACHINE BICEP CURL – Start

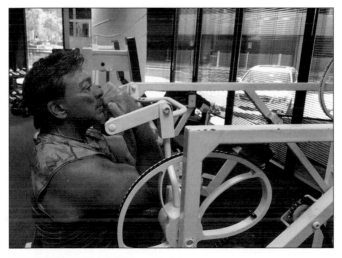

MACHINE BICEP CURL – Finish

TRICEPS ROPE PUSHDOWNS

Rope pushdowns work the triceps, the large muscle on the back of the upper arm. Available in most facilities, a high pulley provides the anchor for a rope that has knobs at both ends. Standing straight up with knees slightly bent and legs slightly apart, start with hands at sternum level in front of you, elbows bent, holding one side of the rope in each hand. Simply push both hands down in front of the body until elbows are straightened out and then slowly raise again to start the next rep. There is no need to spread the hands out at the bottom. This is a common, nonproductive move suggested by many. Continue until posture falters and full extension is no longer attained in good form.

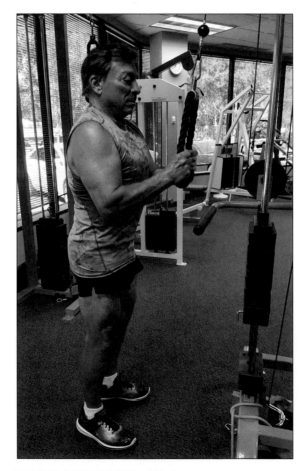

TRICEP PUSHDOWN – Start

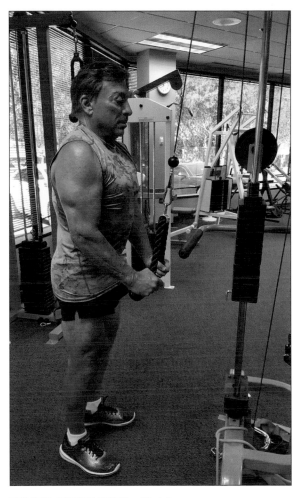

TRICEP PUSHDOWN – Finish

The At-Home Resistance Band SMaRT Workout

If you don't belong to a gym, you can still easily do the SMaRT workout. This program can be performed at home, in the office, or even on the road. You will be using "power bands," which I call "rubber cables." They can be found online and in major sporting goods stores. They come in all sorts of lengths and tension levels, usually with different colors signifying difficulty levels. Make sure you purchase a few different resistance levels, so that you can challenge yourself. I personally prefer sets of cables that provide the following: the capacity to use more than one cable to adjust resistance and a "door stop" knob or knot that can be placed under or in a door jamb when the door is closed, supporting it. It does take some ingenuity to maneuver the bands to work well in providing the appropriate resistance, but with practice you will get the hang of it. As with the weights in the gym section, you will want to choose a resistance that isn't too easy for you but is not so hard that you struggle to complete the full movement.

POWER PAUSE WALL SEATS/SQUATS

The amount of resistance that these large, powerful muscles (legs and hips) require is difficult to attain with rubber cables, so I will recommend a slight twist on the SMaRT principles for this exercise. This exercise works the quadriceps (front of thighs), glutes (butt), and, indirectly, the hamstrings (back of thighs). Start with some heavy duty cables or a combination of strengths, and hold the handles at shoulder height (at sides of shoulders), standing straight up with your back against the wall and both feet securely on top of band(s).You HAVE to hold the handles at shoulder height so that you have tension and it increases as you move from bottom to top. The increased "stretch" of the band as you stand up is what provides the increased tension.

Slowly lower your body by bending the knees until a 90-degree position is reached, as if you are sitting in an imaginary chair against the wall, and hold that position until you start to feel real fatigue in your legs. Now return slowly to the position you started in, standing straight, feeling the resistance increase as you move up and immediately begin to lower your body against the wall. Remember to hold the bottom position (90 degrees) again for a time that produces a serious feeling of fatigue. (The holds will become shorter and shorter as you fatigue the working muscles). This set may take more than 90 seconds due to the isometric or holding segment involved. You'll know you're done when the hold position becomes very shaky and it is almost impossible to return to the start position. Given that, you still don't want to exceed 150 seconds (2½ minutes) in any case.

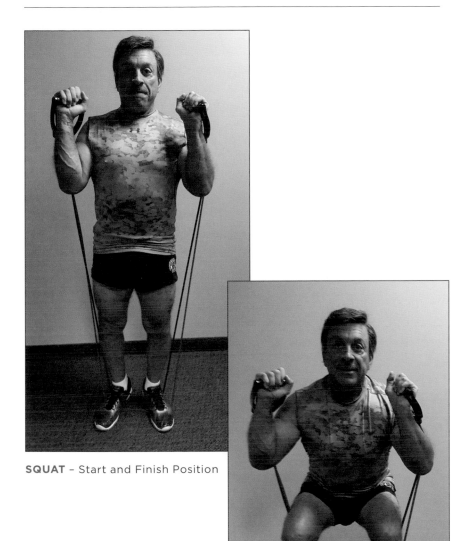

SQUAT – Start and Finish Position

SQUAT – Middle Position

STIFF-LEGGED DEAD LIFTS

This exercise works well for 80 percent of folks. With both feet securely holding the band(s), use a wide leg stand, keeping legs slightly bent (soft knees). Grip the resistance band handles in each hand and slowly raise your torso, focusing on the back of your legs until you are standing up relatively straight with a shoulder "slouch" allowed. Repeat until it becomes difficult to reach finished position in very good form. If your lower back feels achy or resistant during this exercise, don't do it.

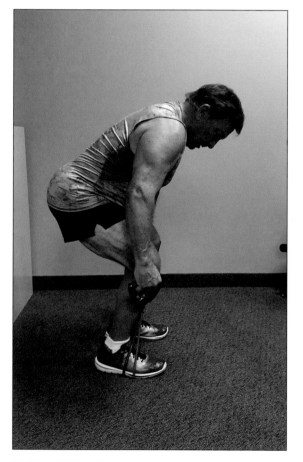

DEAD LIFTS – Start

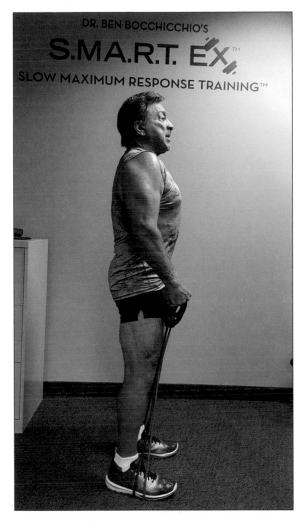

DEAD LIFTS – Finish

ROWING

This exercise works the upper back (trapezius) and mid back (lats). These are huge, powerful muscles. With a door attachment (knob or stopper) securely held by a strong, stable (preferably) locked door at chest height and hands holding handles at shoulder/chest height so that bands are straight out in front of you, slowly pull elbows back, pinching shoulder blades together and keeping elbows "high" at shoulder height, until hands reach just in front of shoulders. Try to "sense" pulling from the back—even though you will feel lots of action in the arms (that's normal). Repeat until no longer able to control the height of your elbows (they will want to "drop") and can no longer reach the finished position with your hands right in front of your shoulders.

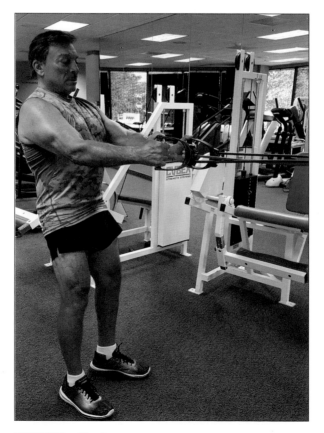

ROWING – Start

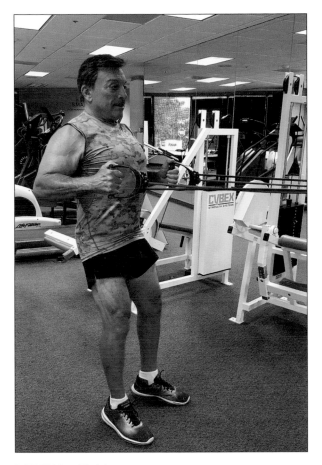

ROWING – Finish

LATERAL RAISES

This exercise works the shoulder muscles and upper back with some arm muscle support required. It can be performed seated or standing. Standing is probably simpler until you become more accustomed to using and stabilizing cables in a seated position. Start standing with your feet slightly apart on the resistance band, your knees slightly bent, and back in a pelvic tilt; your lower back should be slightly rounded not arched and your hands should be at the sides of your thighs, with your knuckles facing out, each hand gripping the handles of the resistance band. Slowly raise both hands (and arms) with slightly bent "soft" elbows directly out to the sides until your arms are 90 degrees (out to shoulder height). Tip: This exercise works "fast twitch" muscle fibers predominantly. What that means is that fatigue usually sets in quickly (from zero to a hundred). One rep might feel manageable and the next one may hit the wall. When your elbows start to bend significantly, and your body wants to bend back, it's over.

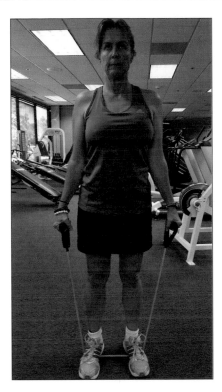

LATERAL RAISE – Start

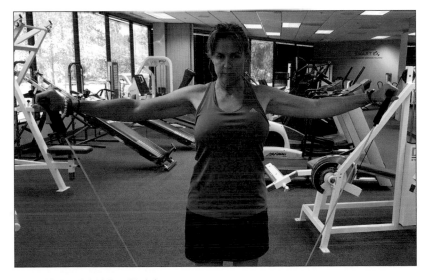

LATERAL RAISE – Finish

PEC/CHEST FLIES

This exercise works the chest (pectoral) muscles and the front (anterior) of the shoulder, with some arm support required. With door attachment (knob or stopper) securely held by strong, stable (preferably) locked door at chest height and hands holding handles at shoulder/chest height with arms out to sides (your back will be to the door, so that the bands are being stretched out behind you), slowly make a big arc with arms remaining at chest/shoulder level so that hands will meet in front of chest at that same height like hugging a tree. The chest muscle goes from the upper arm "through" the front of the shoulder (you will feel this) and ends up on the sternum (the middle of the chest). Repeat until that meeting of the hands (in front of you) becomes difficult enough so that arm and body position move significantly out of form.

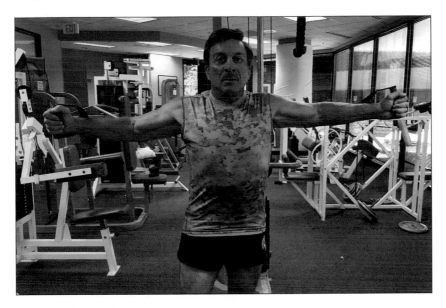

PEC FLIES – Start

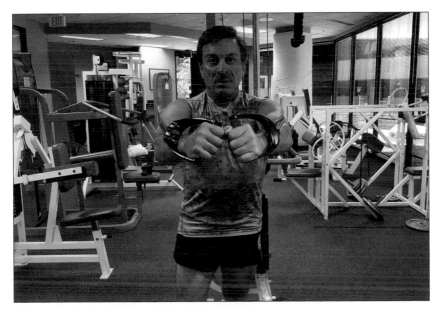

PEC FLIES – Finish

BICEP CURLS

This exercise works the biceps (front of upper arm), forearms, wrists, and hands. There is also major stabilization happening in the abs to maintain proper posture. Start in a standing, secure (posture) position with knees slightly bent and back in a pelvic tilt (lower back slightly rounded but *not* arched). Securely attach the resistance band to something in front of you, so that you can hold the handles and pull back. Extend your arms straight out in front of you at shoulder height, with your palms facing straight up. Slowly bend (do not *pull*) your arms around in an arc, using your elbows as an axel, until your hands reach a position just in front of your shoulders. Slowly return the arms in the same arc that they followed coming forward. Repeat and continue until your body starts to lean back and your hands cannot reach under chin.

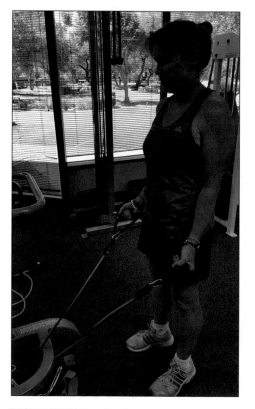

BICEP CURLS – Start

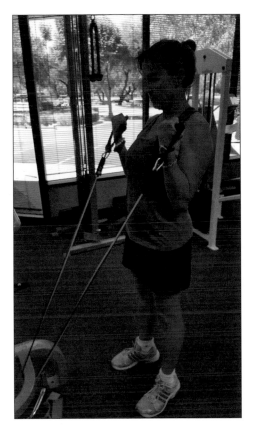

BICEP CURLS – Finish

You can also do the bicep curls standing with cables secured under your feet with a wide stance to take up some slack. Start with arms hanging straight down at sides, gripping handles of resistance band with palms facing forward, and simply bend elbows in and arc until your hands reach your shoulders and return, trying to keep body stationary—not swaying or arching.

TRICEP EXTENSIONS

This exercise works the triceps (back of upper arm) and makes use of abdominals as an important stabilizer group. Secure a band above head height, using the door attachment (knob or stopper) in a strong, stable (preferably) locked door. You want to have a slight angle pulling down. Start with your back to the door and your feet in alternate foot (one in front of the other) position. Grasp the handles of the resistance band and lean forward until you feel stable and balanced and the band is in a stretched position over your head. Slowly pull (although some folks feel a "pushing" move) both of your hands out to a straight arm, extended position. This is another rotary or arching movement. Think of rotating around the axle of your elbows. Continue until your posture becomes inconsistent and you can no longer extend your arms to a finished position.

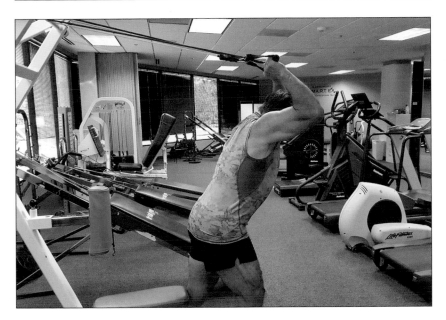

TRICEP EXTENSIONS – Start

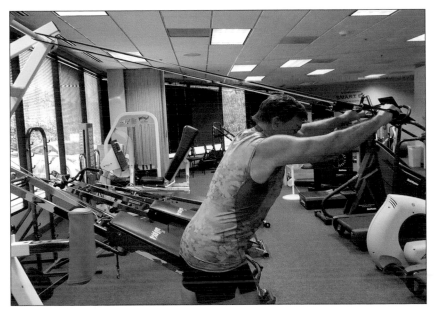

TRICEP EXTENSIONS – Finish

The Total Gym® SMaRT Workout

Total Gym is an exercise machine that has been used in strength training since 1974. It consists of a padded glideboard on an inclined plane and enables users to move with and against gravity, depending upon their position. It engages all muscle groups and can be adjusted to different levels of inclined resistance, using a varied percent of your body weight. Essentially, it provides an entire gym full of equipment in just one machine. Because more than four million people own a Total Gym, it accommodates many different fitness levels, and you can perform exercises for every part of your body. I created a SMaRT workout specifically for it.

As a note of interest, the workout that follows is the exact routine that was used in the 2006 study wherein the average person (50 subjects from 21 to 74, men and women) lost 10 pounds of fat and gained 8 pounds of lean tissue in 10 workouts (5 weeks). The average person lost one third of their body fat in only 10 Total Gym workouts!

LEG PRESSES/SQUATS

This exercise works the quadriceps (front thighs), hamstrings (back of thighs), and "glutes" (butt muscles). Start with your legs bent to 90 degrees, your back supported firmly on the glideboard on a high level, and your feet on the bottom squat stand. Grasp the weight bar with both hands and slowly press upward, sliding the board slowly up to a "not quite" fully extended (straight leg) position and then return (lower) the board to the 90 degree start position. Note: The reason for not straightening the legs to a fully "locked" position is that when the legs "lock," the bones support the weight and the muscles we are trying to tax and "load" constantly can rest. That's why everyone loves this position. It's a *rest* and we don't want the muscle to rest at all until the set (exercise) is completed.

As in all SMaRT exercises, repeat move until you are fatigued and reach a point of muscle failure (incomplete repetition).

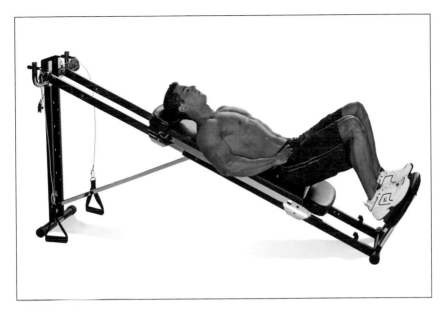

SQUAT – Start

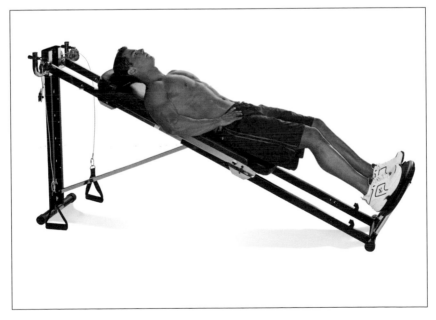

SQUAT – Finish

LYING LEG CURLS

This exercise works the hamstrings (back of thighs) in isolation. I consider this the best leg curl I have ever encountered on any device. It takes the low back and hips out of the precarious position to which they are commonly exposed. Start lying on your back upside down (head facing down) on the glideboard with a slight pelvic tilt (low back pressed "down into bench"); this activates the abdominal muscles and absolutely protects your lower back. Cross your arms against your chest. Bend (drive) heels toward butt as far as your range of motion allows. Think of this movement as a "curl" for your legs and hold the contracted (finished) position for a full second. Repeat until the range of motion is no longer attained and muscles are thoroughly fatigued.

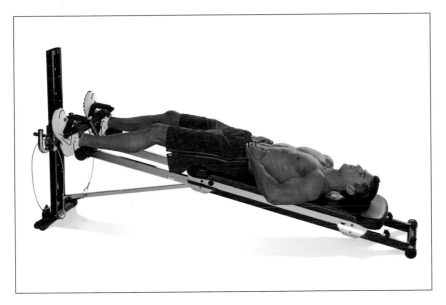

LEG CURL – Start

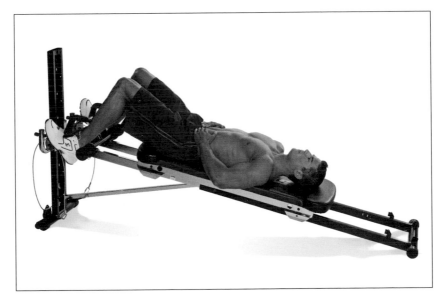

LEG CURL – Finish

GRADED PULL-UPS

This exercise works the large muscles of the upper body (upper and mid back, shoulders, and arms). Lying face down with the top of the glideboard just below chin level and arms extended overhead at about shoulder width, slowly pull up your body until your chin gets past the bar (handle). Continue until you are no longer capable of getting (pulling) your nose up to the bar. The great thing about the Total Gym graded elevation resistance concept is that all people can do some form of a full pull-up by adjusting the elevation.

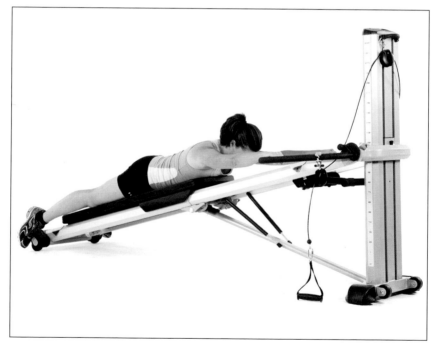

PULL-UP – Start

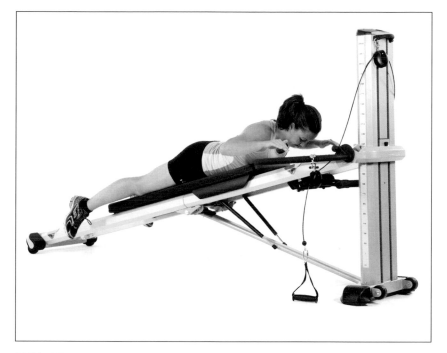

PULL-UP – Finish

PEC (CHEST) FLIES

This exercise works the chest (pectoral) muscle complex and the front of the shoulder. You will also be working your abdomen to ensure good posture. Sitting at the top of the glideboard with your feet crossed or supported on board, arms slightly bent—I call it "long" arms, "soft" elbows)—and hands positioned at shoulder height and out directly to the sides, holding the handles, pull across the body while maintaining arms at shoulder height until your hands touch in front of your chest. Return to original position with arms going out to the sides as far back as you can go without any joint discomfort. When fatigue sets in, the level of the arms and hands drops and the torso starts to "wiggle." STOP. This is an exercise in which form is absolutely vital. If it becomes uncomfortable at any time, either stop and readdress the form or select another exercise (possibly a chest "pressing" move). This will reduce stress on shoulders if they encounter discomfort.

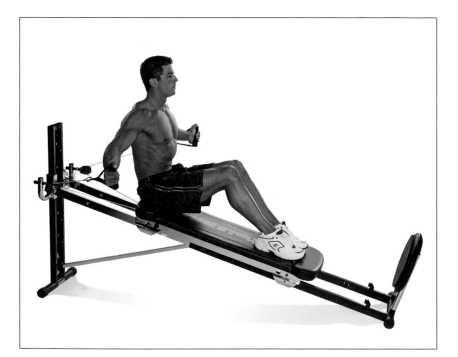

PEC FLY – Start

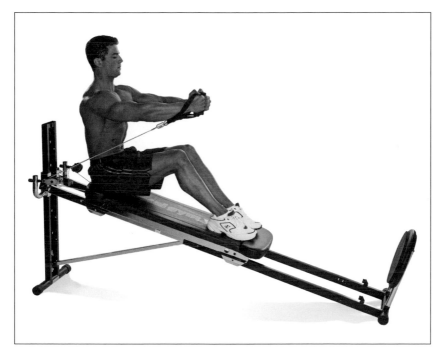

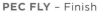

PEC FLY – Finish

DECLINE SHOULDER PRESSES

Again, Total Gym scores high marks for a "different" but incredibly safe and productive "overhead" press movement. It greatly reduces cervical spine (neck) stress and thoroughly works the shoulders, trapezius (shoulder blade area), and triceps. Lying face down with your head inverted on the glideboard, with chin lower than handle (bar), slowly push your body up and away from bottom position to an "almost" full extension, straightening your arms on the way up (don't "lock out") and then return down, bending arms and resisting all the way down to the original start position. Repeat until you are no longer capable of pushing past 90 degrees.

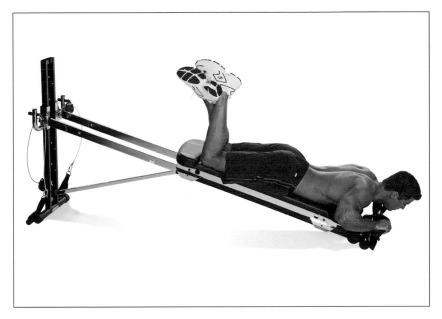

DECLINE SHOULDER PRESS – Start

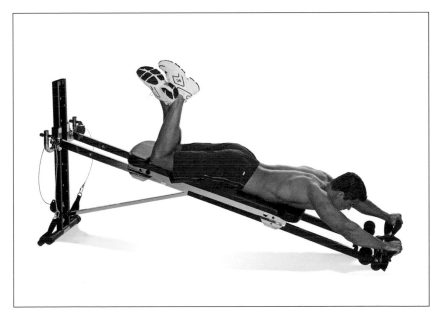

DECLINE SHOULDER PRESS – Finish

SEATED BICEP CURLS

This exercise works the biceps (front of upper arm), forearms, and wrists, as well as the front of your shoulders and abdominal muscles/core for stabilization (posture). Sit up as tall as you can, straddling the glideboard, facing the top of the Total Gym with your arms extended out in front of you at shoulder height and shoulder width apart, with palms facing up. Bend (do not pull) your elbows so that your hands travel in an arc (like a wheel moving around an axle) and your hands finish just under the chin. Return slowly in the same arc until arms get to original extended position at shoulder height and repeat until no longer able to bend past 90 degrees without moving or jerking your body backwards.

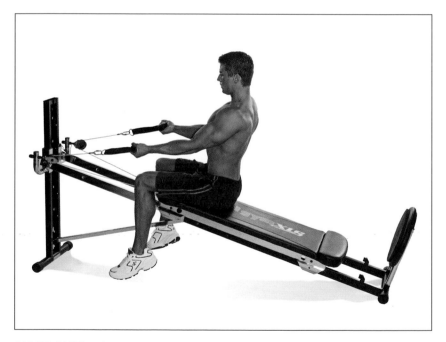

BICEP CURL – Start

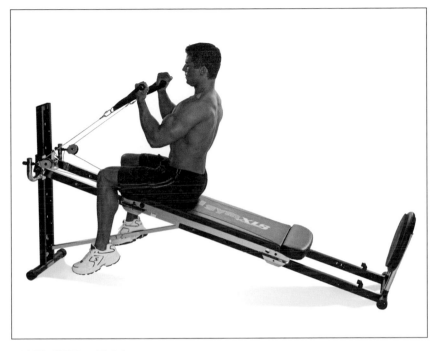

BICEP CURL – Finish

PULL-OVERS

I placed this exercise last in the routine because it thoroughly fin-ishes the job. It works all of the following muscles: abdominals (big time), serratus (rib cage), lats (mid-back), pecs (chest), shoulders, and triceps (back of arms). Lie flat on your back on the glideboard with your knees bent. Start with your arms slightly bent, reach-ing upward (overhead) and holding the handles. Slowly pull (try "feeling" your abs) down in an arc to the front of the thighs, with your shoulders and head lifting up slightly off the board. One of the keys for real productivity is to try to maintain that "pelvic tilt" position, wherein the lower back is pressed into the glideboard at all times. This really activates the abs and protects the lower back from possibility of strain. Repeat until arms "breakdown" (get "shorter") and hands cannot get past the navel (approximately).

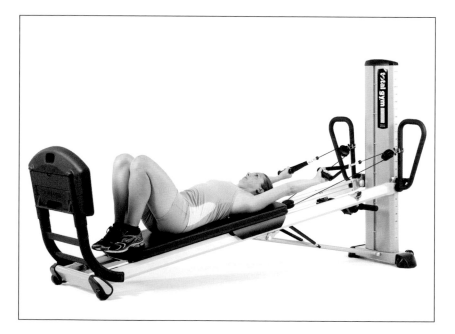

PULL-OVER – Start

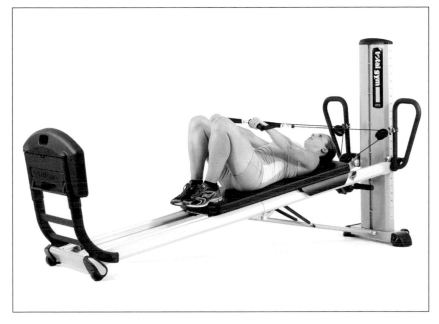

PULL-OVER – Finish

• • •

This is the most important chapter in the five-week metabolic makeover program, because the SMaRT workout utilizes all of your muscles from large to small and activates fat-burning even if you do nothing else. If you solely follow the exercise portion of this program, you will lose fat and gain muscle. For optimal results, however, it does help to follow a diet program that regulates carbohydrates for the reasons we discussed in chapter two. Chapter seven will cover the diet portion of the program, examining the carbohydrate content in certain foods, and offering suggested meal plans and five weeks of menus. But first, since many of you long for the perfect set of abs, I've decided to devote a chapter to the best ab exercises for toning those stubborn muscles. The abs workout is not a necessary part of the SMaRT plan, but since so many people desperately want to lose their gut and tone their abs, I've included it as a bonus in the next chapter for those of you who are interested.

CHAPTER SIX

THE ABS SECRET

What's the secret to great abs? Do you know how many tens of millions of dollars have been sacrificed in this quixotic quest? Too many. I will tell you the truth about the issue. You might not like it, but it will at least save you some money and definitely some time and effort. If you are following the five-week metabolic makeover program, you should be seeing results in your body already. You are beginning to lose fat and gain lean muscle and you likely have more energy. But many of you specifically want toned abdominal muscles, so I wanted to devote a chapter to this tricky, challenging area of the body. This chapter will reveal the real truth about how the abs function, what you may be doing wrong, and the secret for how to exercise so that you really work those abdominal muscles the right way.

The Good—and Bad—News about Abs

I've given this soliloquy thousands of times. "Abs" or abdominal muscles, that six-pack representing extreme fitness and a chance at an underwear modeling career, are a most admired muscular development. If having a perfect set of abs was a common occurrence, however, we would not hold it in such reverence. Unfortunately, most people don't understand how to properly work these muscles, so they spend hours on sit-ups or crunches, never to see the expected result. Here are the real facts, based on anatomy, physiology, and thousands of clinical observations. The Good News: Abdominal muscles are some of the simplest, most responsive muscle groups in the body to effectively work or exercise. The Bad News: You can attain a good degree of muscle function, tone, and development in the abdominal area without *ever* seeing cosmetic evidence of that status. Truthfully, most people don't care about developing strong, functionally healthy abdominal muscles. They want people to *see* their abs! Therein lies the "rub," generating the never-ending journey to six-pack heaven.

Here's why I have deduced that abs are so highly responsive to "proper" exercise. The abdominal wall protects our vital organs. It makes evolutionary sense that these abdominal muscles are important for survival, especially since we walk upright with our bellies exposed. Thus the hyper-responsive, quick adaptation to taxing exercise is a natural consequence of genetic drive.

The Secret: Abs are very simple muscles. Their active job is to round or bend the spine. That's called flexion. Despite some possible protestations from anatomists, that's primarily what abdominal muscles do. They are basically support and stabilizer muscles that are working much of the time, unless we're lying down. However, when they are called upon in a direct, active manner, they get tired quickly and thoroughly. What's the point of this information? Simple: If you are actually working your abdominal muscles directly, they will fatigue quickly and rapidly cease functioning at a high level of demand. Therefore, when people perform huge volumes of reps and sets of "abdominal" exercises, they are almost never, in fact, isolating these most revered of muscle groups. So what are they doing? It *feels* like their abs are working and "burning." However, they are almost always incorporating the hip flexor muscles that bring their thighs back toward the abdominal area. It is extremely hard to sense the difference between these two muscle groups working—until you finally learn how to isolate your abs by using Dr. Ben's Ab Secret.

If you think, as many do, that doing many sets and repetitions in a specific area will create a lean, muscular appearance in that area, then everyone who chewed gum would have the squarest jaw line in the world. Think about it. It doesn't work! Instead, I will show you a couple of exercises that when performed together will work your abdominal muscles better than 100 sit-ups. The great news is that you don't have to complete many reps to obtain real results.

Dr. Ben's Ab Secret

Most people don't realize that if they don't have the right form when performing abdominal exercises, they won't actually be working their abs. So if you do multiple sets of crunches every day the wrong way, you aren't going to see a difference. The two exercises below are the only real way to achieve those six-pack abs. ***Never do any of these exercises if you feel lower back pain at all. Stop immediately!*** You're probably doing them incorrectly and that can be harmful to your lower back.

In my experience, abs are a different animal when it comes to recovery from exercise. I personally do a few reps of Dr. Ben crunches and leg raises every day as part of my morning stretching routine. Note that rounding the back in proper form for isolating abs is also the best stretch for the lower back. In any case, you can exercise your abs more than twice a week if you choose, but please don't fall into the common huge reps and sets trap! Again, "results" will be seen as soon as the fat layer in the lower abdominal area is reduced significantly. That's the catch, and the best exercise for that is done at the table: CUT CARBS!

ABDOMINAL CRUNCHES

Here's a quick Dr. Ben anatomy lesson: Our abdominal muscles are located in "front" of the spine. When they contract, they "round" the spine. This is essentially what they do. ERGO, if your spine is not "rounded," that is, if your back is not pressed against floor (rounded), you are NOT working your abs. So if you find your back straightening whenever you're doing "ab work"—STOP. At this (straightening) point, you will be working your hip flexors, which might feel like ab work, but it is not, and these muscles connect to the lower spine and are the root cause of people hurting their lower backs when attempting ab work.

Lie on your back on the floor, preferably on a carpet, but not on a bed or plush support. Bend your knees to about 90 degrees, with both feet on the floor. Feet should be comfortably apart (usually 6 to 18 inches apart). Roll up a good-sized towel, and place it below your neck. Cross your arms across your chest. Press your lower back down toward the floor, reducing the space between your lower back and the floor. It is *only* in this position—curled, rounded low back—that you can actually isolate and engage the abdominal muscles. If your back is straight, not rounded, your abs cannot be working. That proper rounded position is called a "pelvic tilt."

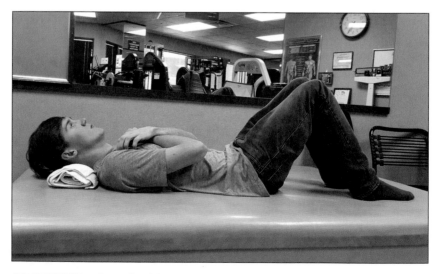

AB CRUNCH – Start Position

Now slowly curl up your torso, raising your chest toward the ceiling or driving your belly button down to the floor. Some people feel like they are trying to press their sternum to their navel. Whatever cue works for you, it is vital to maintain this posture. Curl up as far as you can and when you cease creating movement, try to produce more tension for 3–5 seconds and then slowly return to lying position.

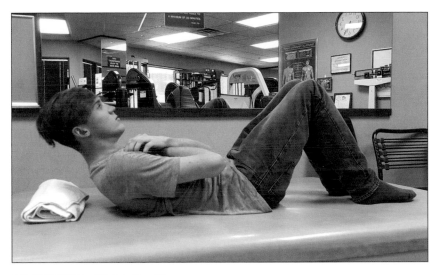

AB CRUNCH – Finish Position

Without resting, repeat repetitions until you can't maintain a significant rounded position. If that position is lost, STOP. At that point, you have ceased working your abs and will engage the hip flexor muscles, which attach to your lower back, and that's how many people injure their lower backs doing "ab" exercises. It's true: isolated ab exercises should *never* hurt your lower back. In fact, they are among the fist exercises I prescribe for most low back rehabs.

If you can do these slow, controlled ab crunches for more than about 90 seconds, you're ready for the most demanding, isolated ab exercise that normal humans can perform. In fact, these are so effective that as few as 3 or 4 repetitions will suffice to drive maximal abdominal muscular development. It is simple but intense and ultimately effective.

LEG RAISES

If you can do these leg raises, you have strong, functionally superior ab muscles, and these exercises will accomplish all that you can reasonably do to develop those prized abdominal muscles. In my experience, you can do these every day as a part of a well-organized stretching routine. Without becoming too technical, contracting abs properly will effectively and safely stretch the opposite (antagonistic) muscle of the problematic lower back area.

The starting position for these leg raises is the end position of the ab crunches: knees bent, arms crossed, and torso crunched or rounded.

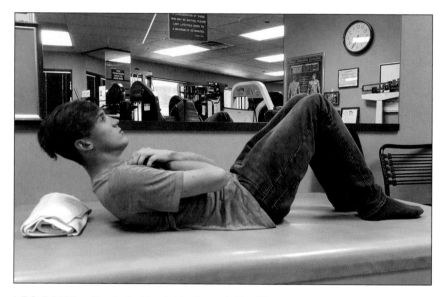

LEG RAISE – Begin in Final Ab Crunch Position

This insures that the back must be rounded and the abs isolated. Now, simply extend and straighten your lower legs, which will now be at a 45 degree angle—half way to perpendicular—to the floor.

Try to keep the lower back rounded, and slowly raise both legs together as high up as you can or until they get to 90 degrees (straight up). Keep legs reasonably straight throughout the movement.

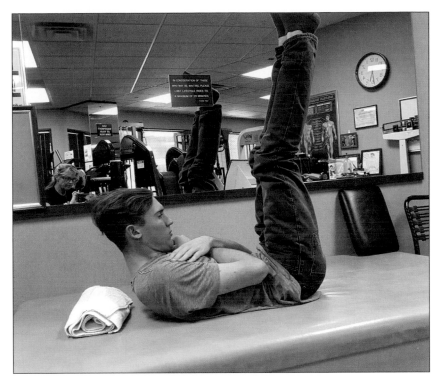

LEG RAISE – Legs-up Active Start Position

Now slowly lower your legs down as far as you can—stop an inch below the floor—without the lower back coming off the floor.

Stay rounded. Most folks can't take the legs down much past 45 degrees to start, so simply do smaller movements and don't try to reach that one inch above the floor position just yet. You will feel your abs working very hard and fatiguing rapidly. When they burn too much or your back loses its flexed, rounded position, STOP. You're done. More is NOT Better! Your range of motion and number of reps will improve, but most very fit people can't do more than 6–10 of these if they do them very slowly, in good form. You'll understand when you do them.

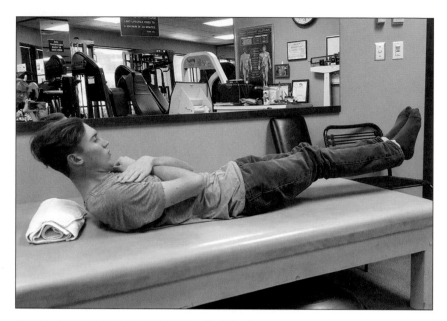

IDEAL ADVANCED LEG RAISE – Finished Position

Fat, Skin, and Diet

Again, many people can attain good tone and decent separation in their abdominal muscles, but very few have the cooperation of extremely low body fat (usually requiring single digit body fat) so that they can really see a six-pack delineation. You also have to be fortunate and young enough to have a good degree of skin tautness (elasticity) in that area to be able to actually *see* that six-pack, defined situation. No amount or volume of ab exercises will enhance the body fat or skin situation. That's just an inane concept upon which purveyors of ab scams thrive. Don't buy it!

Please remember, muscle definition is a state accomplished primarily by two characteristics: The presence of muscle and the absence of fat. One without the other is not going to get you to ab heaven. In simple terms that means that you would be much better served to concentrate on a controlled-carb, fat-burning diet and driving stored fat release through the incorporation of high-intensity muscle work like the SMaRT exercise routine.

Simple observation tells us that people with prominent, "six-pack" abs have a few things in common: youth, leanness, overall muscularity, and taut skin tone. Exercising the abdominal muscles will provide a good basis for one of these components—muscularity. Youth is a very simple circumstance. It really relates to elasticity in the skin and fascia (tissue just beneath the skin). You either have enough to support abdominal definition or you don't. Overall muscularity really depends on body composition (the ratio or percentage of muscle to fat).

One of the best set of abdominal muscles that I have personally encountered was displayed by Pat O'Brien, a college friend and training partner of mine. Pat was a world record holder in the deadlift. Pat NEVER did any ab exercises. He did hugely heavy power lifts, including squats and, most important, deadlifts. In those movements (especially deadlifts), there is a huge stabilizing effort required of the abdominal muscles. They must come into play at enormous intensity to maintain posture and leverage in the spine.

So what's the point of this story? Simply this: In Pat's case, he had youth (he was a grad student in his twenties), he had good skin tone (23 years old), and he was very lean (single digit body fat) with muscular legs and back muscles. He also did only high intensity exercise and very few repetitions. Yet, he had developed world-class abdominals. He didn't need huge numbers of sets and reps, nor did he need specific variations of movements for every segment and function of his abdominals. The point is that neither do you!

• • •

Now you know that you can still have strong, toned abdominal muscles without necessarily seeing a six-pack. Sorry to disappoint you, but at least you no longer have to waste your valuable time doing hundreds of crunches per week to no avail. Remember, with regard to the aesthetic aspects of body shaping, the overall development of the entire muscle structure (head to toe) in a balanced, lean manner will go a long way in producing an admirable physique. If you are a woman who has had kids, it may be tougher for you to achieve high-level definition in your abdominal area (although it is certainly still attainable). For the guys, who tend to deposit some fat in the "love handle" oblique area, doing huge numbers of side bends and twists will do NOTHING to alleviate that problem. Remember the Dr. Ben saying, "If doing huge numbers of repetitions would reduce or tone one specific area, then everyone who chewed gum should have the squarest, most defined jaw line on the planet."

Besides wanting the secret to better abs, people often ask me about the differences between men and women with regard to weight loss. Chapter eight will explore some of these differences, including hormones and metabolism. First I will discuss the SMaRT program for nutrition and diet.

CHAPTER SEVEN

THE SMART EATING PLAN

The foundation of the nutritional component of the SMaRT program is a reduced carbohydrate intake plan. Many popular diets today require you to eliminate multiple food items, such as grains, dairy, sugar, alcohol, legumes, all processed foods, soy, canola oil, mayonnaise, and on and on. It can feel completely overwhelming and unmanageable, especially if you work full time and don't have time to make everything from scratch. The SMaRT Diet is so much easier and far more flexible. While grounded in what our bodies scientifically need from an evolutionary perspective to function in the most optimal way, it also acknowledges that we all live in a modern-day society.

The SMaRT Diet does not force you to give up multiple foods, nor does it even expect you to entirely give up carbohydrates altogether. To be more specific, the plan advised is much lower in carbohydrate content than the average American or modern diet. It is actually a much more rational and biologically compatible plan of healthy eating that corresponds with our genetically dictated physiologic requirements.

There is overwhelming evidence that approximately 80 percent of us have a heightened carbohydrate sensitivity, which means that we have a tendency to respond to eating sugars and starches by storing many of these calories as fat and by becoming insulin resistant.

This combination of chemical responses indicates that cutting down our carbs dramatically may be the best way to stack the metabolic deck in our favor for weight-loss success. Ever mounting scientific evidence indicates that carbohydrates, especially in the form of sugars and simple carbohydrates, are most healthily managed by consuming less of them in our diet. The objective, scientifically sound evidence available suggests that many of our contemporary degenerative disorders are directly linked to the inability to handle the carbohydrate/sugar load imposed by our modern dietary composition. So while many don't need to eliminate them entirely, most of us would be well served to cut back on them dramatically. For example, many people today begin their day with cereal, then have a sandwich on white bread for lunch, and then have pasta or pizza for dinner. Talk about carbohydrate overload! Instead, you want to start incorporating more proteins, fats, and vegetables into your diet. So you could have eggs and bacon for breakfast, a green salad with grilled chicken and avocado for lunch, and a steak with green beans for dinner. It doesn't have to be hard. You can even take a little sugar or honey in your tea or coffee as long as the carb count for the day does not exceed the range that you've chosen.

In my long experience, I have successfully addressed this issue through the application of one of two plans:

1. The initiation phase protocol in which the individual reduces total carbohydrate consumption down to 40 grams per day, and then after some demonstrated acclimatization, a steady but slight bump up of carbohydrate intake is tested.

2. I call this one the "Cold Turkey" approach, which is simply to adhere to a ketogenic diet of only 20 grams of carbs. A ketogenic diet is one that reduces carbs to a point where the body *must* use fat as its primary and preferred fuel source. That chemistry produces molecules called "ketones" and they become primary fuel sources, replacing sugars even in the

brain. This (ketogenic) plan simply eliminates carbs with the exception of some plain, small vegetable dishes and an emphasis on higher, healthy fat foods accompanied by moderate protein eating.

An interesting note on a quick weight-loss plan (if that interests you) is something Dr. Atkins proposed many years ago called a "Fat Fast," which has recently gathered some momentum from scientific interest in it. It is really a form of ketogenic dieting that proposes a daily intake of 1,000 calories composed of 90 percent fat for a short period. This takes some serious organization and menu planning, but you will have the information contained in your menu items to construct a diet for 3 or 4 days each month that contains 90 percent fat, if you choose to try it. Remember, that's most of your calories from fat. It is also suggested on this plan that smaller meals (maybe 4 or 5 a day) might be the best way to go. I have had limited experience with this plan but have seen some significant responses to this unusual method.

(A word of "explanation." Some folks feel that this state of nutritional affairs of practicing a "fat fast" is not healthily sustainable for long periods of time. I have not found this to be a problem, but be advised that this caveat (warning) is sometimes offered).

This chapter will include carb counter charts that you can follow to design the initiation of your carb-controlled diet—(usually) 40 grams maximum per day—or ketogenic diet choices, which should have your daily carbs total even fewer than 40. You can use these charts to help you design your own eating plan, or you can follow the five weeks of menus included for breakfast, lunch, and dinner, and snacks.

While using the meal plans, please remember that you can choose any combination of foods that you like. In other words, if you love certain foods listed on day 10 or 20, you can eat them every day if you like, and if you like a certain breakfast suggestion, you can eat it for any meal—even twice a day! Your main focus should be to reg-ulate (control) carbohydrate intake and make sure to get enough good fat while changing a habit of eating almost exclusively from proteins. Take the time to analyze the composition of the foods you eat using the charts provided. It's actually fun to do. Good luck!

Reading Nutritional Labels

When reading nutritional labels for carbohydrates, it's important to note three items: serving size, number of servings per container, and grams of total carbohydrate per serving. The total carbohy-drate on the label tells you the grams of carbohydrate per serving. Note that there may be more than one serving in the product. If this is the case, you need to multiply the total carbohydrate by the serv-ings per container to get the total carbohydrates in the product—especially if you plan to eat more than one serving.

Sample food label:

Nutrition Facts

Serving Size 1 cup (4 oz)
Serving Per Container 3

Amount Per Serving

Calories 75 Calories from Fat 27

	% Daily Value*
Total Fat 3 g	5%
Saturated Fat 0 g	0%
Cholesterol 0 mg	0%
Sodium 300 mg	4%
Total Carbohydrate 10 g	3%
Dietary Fiber 5 g	20%
Sugars 3 g	
Protein 2 g	

Vitamin A 80% • Vitamin C 60% • Calcium 4% • Iron 4%

* Percent Daily Values are based on a 2,000 calorie diet. Your daily value may be higher or lower depending on your calorie needs:

	Calories:	2,000	2,500
Total Fat	Less than	65g	60g
Sat Fat	Less than	20g	25g
Cholesterol	Less than	300mg	300mg
Sodium	Less than	2,400mg	2,400mg
Total Carbohydrate		300g	375g
Dietary Fiber		25g	30g

Calories per gram:
Fat 9 • Carbohydrate 4 • Protein 4

The serving size for the food is 1 cup.

There are 3 servings or 3 cups in this container.

The total carbohydrate tells how many grams of carbohydrate are in 1 serving.

Sugar is already included in the total carbohydrate amount. This value shows the amount of natural or added sugar.

In the label shown, the serving size is 1 cup, and the number of servings per container is 3. If the total carbohydrates per serving are 10 grams, then the total carbohydrates per container are 30 grams. The total carbohydrate contains all types of carbohydrates, including sugar, so these do not need to be added to the total. Dietary fiber and sugar alcohols (for example, maltitol, sorbitol, xylitol, lactitol) are not completely digested and can be subtracted from the total carbohydrates. The net carbohydrates are 5 grams per serving or 15 grams total per container, because you are subtracting the dietary fibers (5 grams) but not the sugars.

If a food contains ≥5 grams sugar alcohols (which are *not* the same as sugar), half the grams can be subtracted from the "Total Carbohydrate" value. If a food contains ≥5 grams of dietary fiber, half the grams of dietary fiber can be subtracted from the "Total Carbohydrate" value.

Carbohydrate Content in Foods

Most people don't know how many carbohydrates are in certain foods. While we might instinctively know that things like bread and pasta will have more carbs than other foods, most of us don't go around rattling off in our heads how many grams of carbs are in a particular food. Some foods may also be tricky, and you may not realize that they are high in carbohydrates, such as certain fruits and vegetables. For example, an apple has many more carbs than an avocado and a cup of black beans has more carbs than a serving of pancakes. The following tables will help you to see how many carbohydrates are in certain foods—from fruits and vegetables to breads, cereals, and grains—so that you can begin to track how many are in the foods you're eating and adjust your meal plans to remain below 40 grams total per day. In addition, you can use any guide that breaks down foods into their nutrient components and make your individual plan based on tastes and preferences. Find favorites and stick with them.

Carbohydrate Food Tables

In the following tables the amounts given for Calories, Protein, Fat and Carbs are averages. Check the label of the specific product for information.

FOODS WITH LESS THAN 15 CARBS AND NO MORE THAN 10

Food Group	Sub-Group	Food Description	Calories	Protein	Fat	Net Carbs	Serving Size
DAIRY	MILK	BUTTERMILK, CULTURED, LOW-FAT	98	8	2	12	1 CUP
DAIRY	MILK	BUTTERMILK, WHOLE	152	8	8	12	1 CUP
DAIRY	MILK	DRY WHOLE MILK	159	8	9	12	1/4 CUP
DAIRY	MILK	FAT FREE ICE CREAM, NO SUGAR ADDED, FLAVORS OTHER THAN CHOCOLATE	88	3	0	14	1/2 CUP
DAIRY	MILK	GOAT MILK	168	9	10	11	1 CUP
DAIRY	MILK	ICE CREAM, BAR OR STICK, CHOCOLATE COVERED	166	2	12	12	1 BAR
DAIRY	MILK	LOW-FAT MILK, PROTEIN FORTIFIED	118	10	3	14	1 CUP
DAIRY	MILK	MILK, 1% FAT	102	8	2	12	1 CUP
DAIRY	MILK	MILK, IMITATION, NON-SOY	112	4	5	13	1 CUP
DAIRY	MILK	NONFAT MILK	86	8	0	12	1 CUP
DAIRY	MILK	NONFAT MILK, PROTEIN FORTIFIED	101	10	1	14	1 CUP
DAIRY	MILK	WHOLE MILK, 3.25% MILKFAT	149	8	8	12	1 CUP
DAIRY	MILK	YOGURT, FROZEN, FLAVORS NOT CHOCOLATE, NONFAT MILK, WITH LOW-CALORIE SWEETENER	71	3	1	12	1/2 CUP
DAIRY	MILK	YOGURT, VANILLA OR LEMON FLAVOR, NONFAT MILK, SWEETENED WITH LOW-CALORIE SWEETENER	73	7	0	13	6 OZ
FRUITS	FRUIT	APPLES, RAW, GALA, WITH SKIN	62	0	0	12	1 CUP
FRUITS	FRUIT	APPLES, RAW, GOLDEN DELICIOUS, WITH SKIN	62	0	0	12	1 CUP

FOODS WITH LESS THAN 15 CARBS AND NO MORE THAN 10

Food Group	Sub-Group	Food Description	Calories	Protein	Fat	Net Carbs	Serving Size
FRUITS	FRUIT	APPLES, RAW, GRANNY SMITH, WITH SKIN	63	0	0	12	1 CUP
FRUITS	FRUIT	APPLES, RAW, RED DELICIOUS, WITH SKIN	64	0	0	12	1 CUP
FRUITS	FRUIT	APPLES, RAW, WITH SKIN	62	0	0	12	1 CUP
FRUITS	FRUIT	BLUEBERRIES, WILD, FROZEN	80	0	0	13	1 CUP
FRUITS	FRUIT	CHERRIES, SOUR, RED, RAW	52	1	0	11	1 CUP
FRUITS	FRUIT	GRAPEFRUIT, RAW, PINK AND RED AND WHITE	53	1	0	11	1/2 LARGE, (APPROX. 4-1/2" DIA)
FRUITS	FRUIT	MULBERRIES, RAW	60	2	1	12	1 CUP
FRUITS	FRUIT	NECTARINES, RAW	57	1	0	12	1 SMALL, (2-1/3" DIA)
FRUITS	FRUIT	ORANGES, RAW, CALIFORNIA, VALENCIA	59	1	0	11	1 FRUIT, (2-5/8" DIA)
FRUITS	FRUIT	ORANGES, RAW, FLORIDA	65	1	0	13	1 FRUIT, (2-5/8" DIA)
FRUITS	FRUIT	PAPAYAS, RAW	62	1	0	14	1 CUP
FRUITS	FRUIT	PEACHES, RAW	60	1	0	13	1 CUP
FRUITS	FRUIT	POMEGRANATES, RAW	72	1	1	13	1/2 CUP
FRUITS	FRUIT	STRAWBERRIES, RAW	74	2	1	13	1 CUP
FRUITS	FRUIT	WATERMELON, RAW	46	1	0	11	1 CUP
GRAINS	BREAD	BAGELS, CINNAMON-RAISIN	71	3	0	13	1 MINI BAGEL, 2-1/2" DIA
GRAINS	BREAD	BAGELS, EGG	72	3	1	13	1 MINI BAGEL, 2-1/2" DIA
GRAINS	BREAD	BAGELS, OAT BRAN	66	3	0	13	1 MINI BAGEL, 2-1/2" DIA
GRAINS	BREAD	BAGELS, PLAIN (INCLUDES ONION, POPPY, SESAME)	72	3	0	13	1 MINI BAGEL, 2-1/2" DIA
GRAINS	BREAD	BREAD, OAT BRAN	71	3	1	11	1 SLICE

FOODS WITH LESS THAN 15 CARBS AND NO MORE THAN 10

Food Group	Sub-Group	Food Description	Calories	Protein	Fat	Net Carbs	Serving Size
GRAINS	BREAD	BREAD, PITA, WHOLE-WHEAT	74	3	1	13	1 PITA, SMALL 4" DIA
GRAINS	BREAD	BREAD, PUMPERNICKEL	65	2	1	10	1 SLICE
GRAINS	BREAD	BREAD, RYE	82	3	1	13	1 SLICE
GRAINS	BREAD	BREAD, WHEAT	77	3	1	13	1 SLICE
GRAINS	BREAD	BREAD, WHITE	67	2	1	12	1 SLICE
GRAINS	BREAD	BREAD, WHOLE-WHEAT	81	4	1	12	1 SLICE
GRAINS	BREAD	CROISSANTS, BUTTER	114	2	6	12	1 CROISSANT, MINI
GRAINS	BREAD	TORTILLAS, READY-TO-BAKE OR -FRY, CORN	58	1	1	11	1 TORTILLA, APPROX. 6" DIA
GRAINS	CEREAL	CEREALS READY-TO-EAT, RICE, PUFFED, FORTIFIED	56	1	0	13	1 CUP
GRAINS	CEREAL	CEREALS READY-TO-EAT, WHEAT GERM, PLAIN	107	8	3	10	1 OZ
GRAINS	CEREAL GRAINS	WHEAT BRAN, CRUDE	125	9	2	12	1 CUP
GRAINS	COOKIE	COOKIE, WITH PEANUT BUTTER FILLING, CHOCOLATE-COATED	140	2	9	12	2 COOKIES
GRAINS	COOKIE	COOKIES, GRAHAM CRACKERS, PLAIN OR HONEY (INCLUDES CINNAMON)	65	1	2	11	1 CRACKER
GRAINS	COOKIE	COOKIES, OATMEAL, SOFT-TYPE	61	1	2	10	1 COOKIE
GRAINS	COOKIE	COOKIES, VANILLA SANDWICH WITH CRÈME FILLING	72	1	3	11	1 COOKIE
GRAINS	CRACKER	CRACKERS, RYE, WAFERS, SEASONED	84	2	2	11	1 CRACKER, TRIPLE
GRAINS	CRACKER	CRACKERS, STANDARD SNACK-TYPE, REGULAR	82	1	4	10	5 CRACKERS, REGULAR SIZE, ROUND
OTHER	BEVERAGE	BEEF BROTH AND TOMATO JUICE, CANNED	62	1	0	14	1 5-1/2 OZ CAN

FOODS WITH LESS THAN 15 CARBS AND NO MORE THAN 10

Food Group	Sub-Group	Food Description	Calories	Protein	Fat	Net Carbs	Serving Size
OTHER	BEVERAGE	BEVERAGE, COCONUT WATER, READY-TO-DRINK	44	1	0	10	1 CUP
OTHER	BEVERAGE	BEVERAGE, PROTEIN POWDER SOY BASED	175	25	3	10	1 SCOOP
OTHER	BEVERAGE	COCOA MIX, NO SUGAR ADDED, POWDER	72	3	1	13	1 ENVELOPE
OTHER	BEVERAGE	COCOA MIX, WITH ASPARTAME, POWDER, PREPARED WITH WATER	56	2	0	10	6 FL OZ
OTHER	BEVERAGE	LIQUEUR, COFFEE WITH CREAM, 34 PROOF	154	1	7	10	1 JIGGER, 1/2 FL OZ
OTHER	GRAVY	BEEF GRAVY, CANNED, READY-TO-SERVE	123	9	5	10	1 CUP
OTHER	GRAVY	CHICKEN GRAVY, CANNED, READY-TO-SERVE	188	5	14	12	1 CUP
OTHER	GRAVY	MUSHROOM GRAVY, CANNED	119	3	6	12	1 CUP
OTHER	SAUCE	DIP, SALSA CON QUESO, CHEESE AND SALSA, MEDIUM	179	4	12	13	1/2 CUP
OTHER	SNACKS	SNACKS, POTATO CHIPS	157	2	10	14	23 PIECES
OTHER	SNACKS	SNACKS, SESAME STICKS, WHEAT-BASED	151	3	10	12	1 OZ
OTHER	SNACKS	SNACKS, SOY CHIPS OR CRISPS	108	7	2	14	1 OZ
OTHER	SNACKS	SNACKS, SWEET POTATO CHIPS	149	1	9	14	1 OZ
OTHER	SNACKS	SNACKS, TARO CHIPS	115	1	6	14	10 CHIPS
OTHER	SNACKS	SNACKS, TORTILLA CHIPS, LIGHT (BAKED WITH LESS OIL)	74	1	2	11	10 CHIPS
OTHER	SNACKS	SNACKS, VEGETABLE CHIPS, HAIN CELESTIAL GROUP, TERRA CHIPS	145	1	8	13	1 OZ
OTHER	SOUP	BEAN WITH PORK, CANNED SOUP, CONDENSED	168	8	6	14	1/2 CUP
OTHER	SOUP	BEEF AND VEGETABLES, CANNED SOUP, READY-TO-SERVE	120	8	3	12	1 CUP

FOODS WITH LESS THAN 15 CARBS AND NO MORE THAN 10

Food Group	Sub-Group	Food Description	Calories	Protein	Fat	Net Carbs	Serving Size
OTHER	SOUP	CHEESE, CANNED SOUP, CONDENSED	102	1	5	11	1/2 CUP
OTHER	SOUP	CHICKEN AND VEGETABLE, CANNED SOUP, READY-TO-SERVE	84	5	2	10	1 CUP
OTHER	SOUP	CLAM CHOWDER, MANHATTAN, CANNED SOUP, CONDENSED	77	2	2	10	1/2 CUP
OTHER	SOUP	CLAM CHOWDER, NEW ENGLAND, CANNED SOUP, CONDENSED	91	4	3	12	1/2 CUP
OTHER	SOUP	CREAM OF ONION, CANNED SOUP, CONDENSED	111	3	5	12	1/2 CUP
OTHER	SOUP	MINESTRONE, CANNED SOUP, CONDENSED	84	4	3	10	1/2 CUP
OTHER	SOUP	VEGETABLE WITH BEEF BROTH, CANNED SOUP, CONDENSED	81	3	2	11	1/2 CUP
OTHER	SOUP	VEGETARIAN VEGETABLE, CANNED SOUP, CONDENSED	74	2	2	11	1/2 CUP
OTHER	SWEETS	BAKING CHOCOLATE, MEXICAN, SQUARES	85	1	3	14	1 TABLET
OTHER	SWEETS	CANDIES, BUTTERSCOTCH	63	0	1	14	3 PIECES
OTHER	SWEETS	CANDIES, JELLYBEANS	41	0	0	10	10 SMALL
OTHER	SWEETS	CANDIES, MILK CHOCOLATE COATED COFFEE BEANS	154	2	9	13	1 OZ
OTHER	SWEETS	CHOCOLATE, DARK, 70-85% CACAO SOLIDS	167	2	12	10	1 OZ
OTHER	SWEETS	FROZEN NOVELTIES, ICE TYPE, POP	41	0	0	10	1.75 FL OZ POP
OTHER	SWEETS	ICE CREAMS, REGULAR, LOW CARBOHYDRATE, CHOCOLATE	137	2	7	13	1 INDIVIDUAL, (3-1/2 FL OZ)
OTHER	SWEETS	ICE CREAMS, REGULAR, LOW CARBOHYDRATE, VANILLA	143	2	8	12	1/2 CUP
PROTEIN	LEGUME	PEANUTS, SPANISH, OIL-ROASTED	851	41	72	13	1 CUP
PROTEIN	LEGUME	PEANUTS, VALENCIA, OIL-ROASTED	848	39	74	10	1 CUP
PROTEIN	LEGUME	VEGETARIAN STEW	304	42	7	14	1 CUP

FOODS WITH LESS THAN 15 CARBS AND NO MORE THAN 10

Food Group	Sub-Group	Food Description	Calories	Protein	Fat	Net Carbs	Serving Size
PROTEIN	MEAT SUBSTITUTE	VEGETARIAN STEW	304	42	7	14	1 CUP
PROTEIN	NUT	ALMONDS, DRY ROASTED	825	29	73	14	1 CUP
PROTEIN	NUT	ALMONDS, OIL ROASTED	953	33	87	12	1 CUP
PROTEIN	NUT	PINE NUTS, DRIED	909	18	92	13	1 CUP
PROTEIN	SHELLFISH	CRAB, ALASKA KING, IMITATION, MADE FROM SURIMI	81	6	0	13	3 OZ
VEGETABLE	VEGETABLE	BEANS, FAVA, IN POD, RAW	111	10	1	13	1 CUP
VEGETABLE	VEGETABLE	BEANS, LIMA, IMMATURE SEEDS, CANNED, REGULAR PACK, SOLIDS AND LIQUIDS	88	5	0	13	1/2 CUP
VEGETABLE	VEGETABLE	CORN, SWEET, KERNELS ON COB, COOKED	59	2	0	13	1 EAR, YIELDS
VEGETABLE	VEGETABLE	CORN, SWEET, YELLOW, FROZEN, BOILED	65	2	1	13	1/2 CUP
VEGETABLE	VEGETABLE	LEEKS (BULB AND LOWER LEAF-PORTION), RAW	54	1	0	11	1 CUP
VEGETABLE	VEGETABLE	ONIONS, SWEET, RAW	47	1	0	10	1 SERVING
VEGETABLE	VEGETABLE	ONIONS, WHOLE, COOKED	59	1	0	11	1 CUP
VEGETABLE	VEGETABLE	PARSNIPS, COOKED	55	1	0	10	1/2 CUP
VEGETABLE	VEGETABLE	PEAS AND ONIONS, COOKED	81	5	0	12	1 CUP
VEGETABLE	VEGETABLE	PEAS, GREEN, RAW	117	8	1	14	1 CUP
VEGETABLE	VEGETABLE	POTATOES, BAKED, FLESH	57	1	0	12	1/2 CUP
VEGETABLE	VEGETABLE	POTATOES, BAKED, FLESH AND SKIN	57	2	0	12	1/2 CUP
VEGETABLE	VEGETABLE	POTATOES, BOILED, COOKED IN SKIN, FLESH	68	1	0	14	1/2 CUP
VEGETABLE	VEGETABLE	PUMPKIN, CANNED	83	3	1	13	1 CUP
VEGETABLE	VEGETABLE	SOYBEANS, GREEN, COOKED, BOILED	254	22	12	12	1 CUP
VEGETABLE	VEGETABLE	SQUASH, WINTER, ALL VARIETIES, COOKED, BAKED	76	2	1	12	1 CUP

FOODS WITH LESS THAN 10 CARBS AND NO MORE THAN 5

Food Group	Sub-Group	Food Description	Calories	Protein	Fat	Net Carbs	Serving Size
DAIRY	CHEESE	CHEESE, COTTAGE, CREAMED, WITH FRUIT	110	12	4	5	4 OZ
DAIRY	CHEESE	CHEESE, COTTAGE, LOW-FAT, 2% MILKFAT	92	12	3	5	4 OZ
DAIRY	CHEESE	CHEESE, MEXICAN, QUESO CHIHUAHUA	423	24	34	6	1 CUP, CUBED
DAIRY	CHEESE	CHEESE, SWISS	502	36	37	7	1 CUP, CUBED
DAIRY	MILK	CREAM, HEAVY WHIPPING	821	5	88	7	1 CUP, YIELDS 2 CUPS WHIPPED
DAIRY	MILK	CREAM, SOUR, CULTURED	444	5	45	7	1 CUP
DAIRY	MILK	YOGURT, GREEK, PLAIN, NONFAT	100	17	1	6	1 CONTAINER
DAIRY	MILK	YOGURT, PLAIN, WHOLE MILK, 8 GRAMS PROTEIN PER 8 OUNCE	104	6	6	8	6 OZ
FATS & OILS	DRESSING	SALAD DRESSING, HONEY MUSTARD	139	0	12	7	2 TBSP.
FATS & OILS	DRESSING	SALAD DRESSING, POPPY SEED, CREAMY	132	0	11	8	2 TBSP.
FATS & OILS	DRESSING	SALAD DRESSING, RUSSIAN DRESSING	53	0	4	5	1 TBSP.
FRUITS	FRUIT	AVOCADOS, RAW, FLORIDA	276	5	23	5	1 CUP
FRUITS	FRUIT	BLACKBERRIES, RAW	62	2	1	6	1 CUP
FRUITS	FRUIT	BLUEBERRIES, RAW	39	1	0	8	50 BERRIES
FRUITS	FRUIT	CLEMENTINE, RAW	35	1	0	8	1 FRUIT
FRUITS	FRUIT	CRANBERRIES, RAW	46	0	0	7	1 CUP
FRUITS	FRUIT	FIGS, RAW	37	0	0	9	1 MEDIUM, (2-1/4" DIA)
FRUITS	FRUIT	GRAPES, RED OR GREEN (EUROPEAN TYPE, SUCH AS THOMPSON SEEDLESS), RAW	34	0	0	9	10 GRAPES
FRUITS	FRUIT	LIMES, RAW	20	0	0	5	1 FRUIT, (2" DIA)
FRUITS	FRUIT	MELONS, CASABA, RAW	48	2	0	9	1 CUP

FOODS WITH LESS THAN 10 CARBS AND NO MORE THAN 5

Food Group	Sub-Group	Food Description	Calories	Protein	Fat	Net Carbs	Serving Size
FRUITS	FRUIT	PEARS, ASIAN, RAW	51	1	0	9	1 FRUIT, 2-1/4" HIGH × 2-1/2" DIA
FRUITS	FRUIT	PLUMS, RAW	30	0	0	7	1 FRUIT, (2-1/8" DIA)
FRUITS	FRUIT	PRICKLY PEARS, RAW	61	1	1	9	1 CUP
FRUITS	FRUIT	RASPBERRIES, RAW	64	1	1	7	1 CUP
FRUITS	FRUIT	TANGERINES (MANDARIN ORANGES), RAW	40	1	0	9	1 SMALL, (2-1/4" DIA)
FRUITS	JUICE	PRUNE JUICE, CANNED	23	0	0	6	1 FL OZ
GRAINS	BREAD	BREAD, MULTI-GRAIN (INCLUDES WHOLE-GRAIN)	69	3	1	9	1 SLICE
GRAINS	BREAD	BREAD, WHEAT, WHITE WHEAT	67	3	1	9	1 SLICE
GRAINS	BREAD	TACO SHELLS, BAKED	61	1	3	7	1 MEDIUM, APPROX. 5" DIA
GRAINS	BREAD	TOSTADA SHELLS, CORN	57	1	3	7	1 PIECE
GRAINS	CEREAL	CEREALS READY-TO-EAT, WHEAT, PUFFED, FORTIFIED	44	2	0	9	1 CUP
GRAINS	CEREAL GRAINS	CORN BRAN, CRUDE	170	6	1	5	1 CUP
GRAINS	COOKIE	COOKIES, CHOCOLATE CHIP, SOFT-TYPE	62	1	3	9	1 COOKIE
GRAINS	COOKIE	COOKIES, FORTUNE	30	0	0	7	1 COOKIE
GRAINS	COOKIE	COOKIES, GINGERSNAPS	29	0	1	5	1 COOKIE
GRAINS	COOKIE	COOKIES, PEANUT BUTTER SANDWICH, REGULAR	67	1	3	9	1 COOKIE
GRAINS	COOKIE	COOKIES, PEANUT BUTTER, SOFT-TYPE	69	1	4	9	1 COOKIE
GRAINS	CRACKER	CRACKERS, MULTIGRAIN	67	1	3	9	4 CRACKERS
GRAINS	CRACKER	CRACKERS, WHEAT, REGULAR	66	1	2	9	2 CRACKERS
GRAINS	SNACKS	SNACKS, POPCORN, CAKES	38	1	0	8	1 CAKE

FOODS WITH LESS THAN 10 CARBS AND NO MORE THAN 5

Food Group	Sub-Group	Food Description	Calories	Protein	Fat	Net Carbs	Serving Size
GRAINS	SNACKS	SNACKS, POPCORN, CHEESE-FLAVOR	58	1	4	5	1 CUP
OTHER	BEVERAGE	BEVERAGE, ENERGY DRINK, SUGAR-FREE WITH GUARANA	19	0	0	5	16 FL OZ
OTHER	BEVERAGE	WINE, TABLE, RED, BURGUNDY	127	0	0	5	5 FL OZ
OTHER	BEVERAGE	WINE, TABLE, WHITE, CHENIN BLANC	118	0	0	5	5 FL OZ
OTHER	BEVERAGE	WINE, TABLE, WHITE, RIESLING	118	0	0	6	5 FL OZ
OTHER	SAUCE	BARBECUE SAUCE	29	0	0	7	1 TBSP.
OTHER	SAUCE	HOISIN SAUCE, READY-TO-SERVE	35	1	1	7	1 TBSP.
OTHER	SAUCE	PASTA SAUCE, SPAGHETTI/MARINARA, READY-TO-SERVE, LOW SODIUM	65	2	2	8	1/2 CUP
OTHER	SAUCE	SALSA SAUCE, READY-TO-SERVE	38	2	0	7	1/2 CUP
OTHER	SAUCE	SHRIMP COCKTAIL SAUCE, READY-TO-SERVE	30	0	0	8	2 TBSP.
OTHER	SAUCE	STEAK SAUCE, TOMATO BASED	32	0	0	6	2 TBSP.
OTHER	SOUP	BEEF MUSHROOM, CANNED SOUP, CONDENSED	77	6	3	7	1/2 CUP
OTHER	SOUP	BEEF NOODLE, CANNED SOUP, CONDENSED	84	5	3	8	1/2 CUP
OTHER	SOUP	BROCCOLI CHEESE, CANNED SOUP, CONDENSED	105	3	6	7	1/2 CUP
OTHER	SOUP	CHICKEN NOODLE, CANNED SOUP, CONDENSED	60	3	2	7	1/2 CUP
OTHER	SOUP	CHICKEN VEGETABLE, CANNED SOUP, CONDENSED	74	4	3	7	1/2 CUP
OTHER	SOUP	CREAM OF CELERY, CANNED SOUP, CONDENSED	91	2	6	8	1/2 CUP
OTHER	SOUP	CREAM OF CHICKEN, CANNED SOUP, CONDENSED	113	3	7	9	1/2 CUP

FOODS WITH LESS THAN 10 CARBS AND NO MORE THAN 5

Food Group	Sub-Group	Food Description	Calories	Protein	Fat	Net Carbs	Serving Size
OTHER	SOUP	CREAM OF MUSHROOM, CANNED SOUP, CONDENSED	100	2	7	8	1/2 CUP
OTHER	SOUP	ONION SOUP, DRY, MIX	21	1	0	5	1 TBSP.
OTHER	SOUP	ONION, CANNED SOUP, CONDENSED	57	4	2	7	1/2 CUP
OTHER	SOUP	VEGETABLE BEEF, CANNED SOUP, CONDENSED	79	6	2	8	1/2 CUP
OTHER	SPICES AND HERBS	GARLIC POWDER	32	2	0	6	1 TBSP.
OTHER	SWEETS	CANDIES, CARAMELS	39	0	1	8	1 PIECE
OTHER	SWEETS	CANDIES, HARD	24	0	0	6	1 PIECE
OTHER	SWEETS	CANDIES, SEMISWEET CHOCOLATE	67	1	4	8	1 SERVING
OTHER	SWEETS	FROZEN NOVELTIES, JUICE TYPE, ORANGE	28	0	0	7	1 FL OZ
OTHER	SWEETS	FRUIT BUTTERS, APPLE	29	0	0	7	1 TBSP.
OTHER	SWEETS	JAMS AND PRESERVES, DIETETIC (WITH SODIUM SACCHARIN), ANY FLAVOR	18	0	0	8	1 TBSP.
OTHER	SWEETS	JELLIES, REDUCED SUGAR, HOME PRESERVED	34	0	0	9	1 TBSP.
OTHER	SWEETS	PUDDINGS, CHOCOLATE, READY-TO-EAT	40	1	1	6	1 OZ
OTHER	SWEETS	PUDDINGS, VANILLA, READY-TO-EAT	36	0	1	6	1 OZ
OTHER	SWEETS	SYRUPS, DIETETIC	6	0	0	7	1 TBSP.
PROTEIN	CHICKEN	CHICKEN PATTY, FROZEN, COOKED	172	9	12	8	1 PATTY
PROTEIN	FISH	FISH STICKS, FROZEN, PREPARED	78	3	5	6	1 STICK, (4" × 1" × 1/2")
PROTEIN	FISH	TUNA SALAD	159	14	8	8	3 OZ
PROTEIN	LEGUME	PEANUT BUTTER, SMOOTH STYLE	191	7	16	5	2 TBSP.
PROTEIN	LEGUME	PEANUTS, ALL TYPES, OIL-ROASTED	863	40	76	8	1 CUP

FOODS WITH LESS THAN 10 CARBS AND NO MORE THAN 5

Food Group	Sub-Group	Food Description	Calories	Protein	Fat	Net Carbs	Serving Size
PROTEIN	LEGUME	SOY PROTEIN CONCENTRATE	93	16	0	7	1 OZ
PROTEIN	LEGUME	SOY PROTEIN CONCENTRATE, CRUDE PROTEIN BASIS (N X 6.25), PRODUCED BY ACID WASH	92	18	0	5	1 OZ
PROTEIN	LEGUME	SOYBEANS, MATURE COOKED, BOILED	298	29	15	7	1 CUP
PROTEIN	LUNCH MEAT	MEATBALLS, FROZEN, ITALIAN STYLE	243	12	19	5	3 OZ
PROTEIN	LUNCH MEAT	SOYBEANS, MATURE SEEDS, SPROUTED, COOKED, STEAMED	76	8	4	5	1 CUP
PROTEIN	MEAT SUBSTITUTE	BACON, MEATLESS	446	15	43	5	1 CUP
PROTEIN	MEAT SUBSTITUTE	FRANKFURTER, MEATLESS	326	27	19	6	1 CUP
PROTEIN	MEAT SUBSTITUTE	MEATBALLS, MEATLESS	284	30	13	5	1 CUP
PROTEIN	MEAT SUBSTITUTE	VEGGIE BURGERS OR SOY BURGERS, UNPREPARED	124	11	4	7	1 PATTIE
PROTEIN	NUT	CASHEW NUTS, DRY ROASTED	163	4	13	8	1 OZ
PROTEIN	NUT	COCONUT MEAT, RAW	283	3	27	5	1 CUP
PROTEIN	NUT	COCONUT MILK, RAW (LIQUID EXPRESSED FROM GRATED MEAT AND WATER)	552	5	57	8	1 CUP
PROTEIN	NUT	COCONUT WATER (LIQUID FROM COCONUTS)	46	2	0	6	1 CUP
PROTEIN	NUT	HAZELNUTS OR FILBERTS	722	17	70	8	1 CUP
PROTEIN	NUT	MACADAMIA NUTS, DRY ROASTED	948	10	100	7	1 CUP
PROTEIN	NUT	PISTACHIO NUTS, DRY ROASTED	160	6	13	5	1 OZ, (49 KERNELS)
PROTEIN	NUT	WALNUTS, ENGLISH	765	18	76	8	1 CUP
PROTEIN	SAUSAGE	SAUSAGE, CHICKEN, BEEF, PORK, SKINLESS, SMOKED	181	11	12	7	1 LINK
PROTEIN	SEAFOOD	ABALONE, MIXED SPECIES, FRIED	161	17	6	9	3 OZ

FOODS WITH LESS THAN 10 CARBS AND NO MORE THAN 5

Food Group	Sub-Group	Food Description	Calories	Protein	Fat	Net Carbs	Serving Size
PROTEIN	SEAFOOD	MUSSEL, BLUE	146	20	4	6	3 OZ
PROTEIN	SEAFOOD	OYSTER, EASTERN	67	6	2	6	3 OZ
PROTEIN	SEAFOOD	OYSTER, EASTERN, WILD	87	10	3	5	3 OZ
PROTEIN	SEAFOOD	OYSTER, PACIFIC	139	16	4	8	3 OZ
PROTEIN	SEAFOOD	SCALLOP (BAY AND SEA), STEAMED	94	17	1	5	3 OZ
VEGETABLE	VEGETABLE	BEANS, SNAP, GREEN, COOKED	38	2	0	5	1 CUP
VEGETABLE	VEGETABLE	BEANS, SNAP, YELLOW, COOKED	38	2	0	5	1 CUP
VEGETABLE	VEGETABLE	BEETS, CANNED, DRAINED SOLIDS	49	1	0	8	1 CUP
VEGETABLE	VEGETABLE	BEETS, COOKED, BOILED	37	1	0	6	1/2 CUP
VEGETABLE	VEGETABLE	BEETS, RAW	58	2	0	9	1 CUP
VEGETABLE	VEGETABLE	BRUSSELS SPROUTS, COOKED	65	6	1	7	1 CUP
VEGETABLE	VEGETABLE	BRUSSELS SPROUTS, RAW	38	3	0	5	1 CUP
VEGETABLE	VEGETABLE	CARROTS, RAW	52	1	0	8	1 CUP
VEGETABLE	VEGETABLE	CATSUP	17	0	0	5	1 TBSP.
VEGETABLE	VEGETABLE	EDAMAME, FROZEN, PREPARED	189	17	8	7	1 CUP
VEGETABLE	VEGETABLE	EGGPLANT, COOKED	35	1	0	7	1 CUP
VEGETABLE	VEGETABLE	KOHLRABI, COOKED	48	3	0	9	1 CUP
VEGETABLE	VEGETABLE	MUSHROOMS, SHIITAKE, COOKED	40	1	0	8	4 MUSHROOMS
VEGETABLE	VEGETABLE	MUSHROOMS, WHITE, COOKED	44	3	1	5	1 CUP
VEGETABLE	VEGETABLE	ONIONS, RAW	46	1	0	9	1 CUP
VEGETABLE	VEGETABLE	ONIONS, YELLOW, SAUTÉED	115	1	9	6	1 CUP
VEGETABLE	VEGETABLE	PEAS AND CARROTS, COOKED	38	2	0	6	1/2 CUP
VEGETABLE	VEGETABLE	PEAS, EDIBLE-PODDED, COOKED	80	6	1	8	1 CUP

FOODS WITH LESS THAN 10 CARBS AND NO MORE THAN 5

Food Group	Sub-Group	Food Description	Calories	Protein	Fat	Net Carbs	Serving Size
VEGETABLE	VEGETABLE	PEAS, GREEN, CANNED, DRAINED SOLIDS	59	4	0	8	1/2 CUP
VEGETABLE	VEGETABLE	PEAS, GREEN, COOKED	62	4	0	7	1/2 CUP
VEGETABLE	VEGETABLE	PEPPERS, HOT CHILI, GREEN, RAW	30	2	0	6	1/2 CUP
VEGETABLE	VEGETABLE	PEPPERS, HOT CHILI, RED, RAW	30	1	0	6	1/2 CUP
VEGETABLE	VEGETABLE	PEPPERS, SWEET, GREEN, COOKED	38	1	0	7	1 CUP
VEGETABLE	VEGETABLE	PEPPERS, SWEET, RED, COOKED	38	1	0	7	1 CUP
VEGETABLE	VEGETABLE	PEPPERS, SWEET, RED, RAW	46	1	0	6	1 CUP
VEGETABLE	VEGETABLE	PICKLE RELISH, HAMBURGER	19	0	0	5	1 TBSP.
VEGETABLE	VEGETABLE	PICKLE RELISH, SWEET	20	0	0	5	1 TBSP.
VEGETABLE	VEGETABLE	PIMENTO, CANNED	44	2	1	6	1 CUP
VEGETABLE	VEGETABLE	POTATOES, BOILED, COOKED IN SKIN, SKIN	27	1	0	5	1 SKIN
VEGETABLE	VEGETABLE	POTATOES, FRENCH FRIED, SHOESTRING	50	1	2	7	10 STRIP
VEGETABLE	VEGETABLE	POTATOES, HASH BROWN, FROZEN, PLAIN, PREPARED, PAN FRIED IN CANOLA OIL	64	1	3	7	1 PATTY, OVAL (APPROX. 3″ × 1-1/2″ × 1/2″)
VEGETABLE	VEGETABLE	SQUASH, SUMMER, ALL VARIETIES, COOKED, BOILED	36	2	1	5	1 CUP
VEGETABLE	VEGETABLE	SQUASH, WINTER, ALL VARIETIES, RAW	39	1	0	8	1 CUP
VEGETABLE	VEGETABLE	TOMATO PRODUCTS, CANNED, SAUCE	59	3	1	9	1 CUP
VEGETABLE	VEGETABLE	TOMATO SAUCE, CANNED	59	3	1	9	1 CUP
VEGETABLE	VEGETABLE	TOMATOES, CRUSHED, CANNED	39	2	0	7	1/2 CUP
VEGETABLE	VEGETABLE	TOMATOES, GREEN, RAW	42	2	0	7	1 LARGE
VEGETABLE	VEGETABLE	TOMATOES, RED, RAW	32	2	0	5	1 CUP

FOODS WITH LESS THAN 10 CARBS AND NO MORE THAN 5

Food Group	Sub-Group	Food Description	Calories	Protein	Fat	Net Carbs	Serving Size
VEGETABLE	VEGETABLE	TURNIPS, COOKED, BOILED	51	2	0	7	1 CUP
VEGETABLE	VEGETABLE	TURNIPS, RAW	36	1	0	6	1 CUP
VEGETABLE	VEGETABLE	WATER CHESTNUTS, CHINESE, CANNED, SOLIDS AND LIQUIDS	35	1	0	7	1/2 CUP
VEGETABLE	VEGETABLE	YAM BEAN (JICAMA), RAW	49	1	0	5	1 CUP
VEGETABLE	VEGETABLE JUICE	VEGETABLE JUICE COCKTAIL, CANNED	56	2	1	9	1 CUP
VEGETABLE	VEGETABLE JUICE	VEGETABLE JUICE COCKTAIL, LOW SODIUM, CANNED	35	2	1	6	6 FL OZ

FOODS WITH LESS THAN 5 CARBS AND NO MORE THAN 1

Food Group	Sub Group	Food Description	Calories	Protein	Fat	Net Carbs	Serving Size
DAIRY	CHEESE	CHEESE, BLUE	99	6	8	1	1 OZ
DAIRY	CHEESE	CHEESE, CARAWAY	105	7	8	1	1 OZ
DAIRY	CHEESE	CHEESE, CHEDDAR	110	7	9	2	1 OZ
DAIRY	CHEESE	CHEESE, CHEDDAR OR COLBY LOW-SODIUM	450	28	37	2	1 CUP, CUBED
DAIRY	CHEESE	CHEESE, COLBY	440	28	36	4	4 OZ
DAIRY	CHEESE	CHEESE, COTTAGE, CREAMED, LARGE OR SMALL CURD	111	13	5	4	4 OZ
DAIRY	CHEESE	CHEESE, CREAM	48	1	5	1	1 TBSP.
DAIRY	CHEESE	CHEESE, FETA	75	4	6	1	1 OZ
DAIRY	CHEESE	CHEESE, FONTINA	420	28	34	2	1 CUP
DAIRY	CHEESE	CHEESE, FRESH, QUESO FRESCO	365	22	29	4	1 CUP
DAIRY	CHEESE	CHEESE, GOAT, HARD TYPE	127	9	10	1	1 OZ
DAIRY	CHEESE	CHEESE, GOUDA	100	7	8	1	1 OZ

FOODS WITH LESS THAN 5 CARBS AND NO MORE THAN 1

Food Group	Sub Group	Food Description	Calories	Protein	Fat	Net Carbs	Serving Size
DAIRY	CHEESE	CHEESE, MEXICAN, QUESO ANEJO	106	6	8	1	1 OZ
DAIRY	CHEESE	CHEESE, MEXICAN, QUESO ASADERO	402	26	32	3	1 CUP, CUBED
DAIRY	CHEESE	CHEESE, MONTEREY	421	28	34	1	1 CUP, CUBED
DAIRY	CHEESE	CHEESE, MOZZARELLA, LOW SODIUM	316	31	19	4	1 CUP, CUBED
DAIRY	CHEESE	CHEESE, MOZZARELLA, PART SKIM MILK	71	7	4	1	1 OZ
DAIRY	CHEESE	CHEESE, MOZZARELLA, WHOLE MILK	85	6	6	1	1 OZ
DAIRY	CHEESE	CHEESE, MUENSTER	416	26	34	1	1 CUP, CUBED
DAIRY	CHEESE	CHEESE, NEUFCHATEL	71	3	6	1	1 OZ
DAIRY	CHEESE	CHEESE, PARMESAN, GRATED	21	1	1	1	1 TBSP.
DAIRY	CHEESE	CHEESE, PARMESAN, HARD	110	10	7	1	1 OZ
DAIRY	CHEESE	CHEESE, PASTEURIZED PROCESS, AMERICAN	102	5	9	1	1 OZ
DAIRY	CHEESE	CHEESE, PASTEURIZED PROCESS, CHEDDAR OR AMERICAN, LOW SODIUM	425	25	35	2	1 CUP, CUBED
DAIRY	CHEESE	CHEESE, PROVOLONE	100	7	8	1	1 OZ
DAIRY	CHEESE	CHEESE, RICOTTA, PART SKIM MILK	39	3	2	1	1 OZ
DAIRY	CHEESE	CHEESE, RICOTTA, WHOLE MILK	216	14	16	4	1/2 CUP
DAIRY	CHEESE	CHEESE, ROMANO	108	9	8	1	1 OZ
DAIRY	CHEESE	CHEESE, ROQUEFORT	103	6	9	1	1 OZ
DAIRY	MILK	CHOCOLATE MILK, WHOLE	26	1	1	3	1 FL OZ
DAIRY	MILK	CREAM, HALF AND HALF	20	0	2	1	1 TBSP.
DAIRY	MILK	SOUR DRESSING, NON-BUTTERFAT, CULTURED, FILLED CREAM-TYPE	21	0	2	1	1 TBSP.
FATS & OILS	DRESSING	CREAMY DRESSING, MADE WITH SOUR CREAM AND/OR BUTTERMILK AND OIL, REDUCED CALORIE	24	0	2	1	1 TBSP.

FOODS WITH LESS THAN 5 CARBS AND NO MORE THAN 1

Food Group	Sub Group	Food Description	Calories	Protein	Fat	Net Carbs	Serving Size
FATS & OILS	DRESSING	SALAD DRESSING, BLUE OR ROQUEFORT CHEESE DRESSING	73	0	8	1	1 TBSP.
FATS & OILS	DRESSING	SALAD DRESSING, COLESLAW	62	0	5	4	1 TBSP.
FATS & OILS	DRESSING	SALAD DRESSING, FRENCH DRESSING	73	0	7	2	1 TBSP.
FATS & OILS	DRESSING	SALAD DRESSING, GREEN GODDESS	64	0	6	1	1 TBSP.
FATS & OILS	DRESSING	SALAD DRESSING, ITALIAN DRESSING	41	0	4	1	1 TBSP.
FATS & OILS	DRESSING	SALAD DRESSING, MAYONNAISE TYPE	35	0	3	2	1 TBSP.
FATS & OILS	DRESSING	SALAD DRESSING, RANCH DRESSING	63	0	7	1	1 TBSP.
FATS & OILS	DRESSING	SALAD DRESSING, SESAME SEED DRESSING	66	0	7	1	1 TBSP.
FATS & OILS	DRESSING	SALAD DRESSING, SWEET AND SOUR	2	0	0	1	1 TBSP.
FATS & OILS	DRESSING	SALAD DRESSING, THOUSAND ISLAND	61	0	6	2	1 TBSP.
FRUITS	FRUIT	APRICOTS, DRIED, SULFURED, UNCOOKED	8	0	0	2	1 HALF
FRUITS	FRUIT	AVOCADOS, RAW, CALIFORNIA	384	5	35	4	1 CUP
FRUITS	FRUIT	DATES, DEGLET NOOR	20	0	0	4	1 FRUIT
FRUITS	FRUIT	FIGS, DRIED, UNCOOKED	21	0	0	4	1 FIG
FRUITS	FRUIT	LEMONS, RAW, WITHOUT PEEL	17	1	0	3	1 FRUIT, (2-1/8" DIA)
FRUITS	FRUIT	OLIVES, RIPE, CANNED	23	0	2	1	1 OZ
FRUITS	FRUIT	OLIVES, RIPE, CANNED SUPER COLOSSAL	12	0	1	1	1 SUPER COLOSSAL
FRUITS	FRUIT	ORANGE PEEL, RAW	6	0	0	1	1 TBSP.
FRUITS	FRUIT	RHUBARB, RAW	26	1	0	4	1 CUP
FRUITS	JUICE	LEMON JUICE, CANNED OR BOTTLED	3	0	0	1	1 TBSP.
FRUITS	JUICE	LEMON JUICE, FROZEN, UNSWEETENED, SINGLE STRENGTH	7	0	0	2	1 FL OZ

FOODS WITH LESS THAN 5 CARBS AND NO MORE THAN 1

Food Group	Sub Group	Food Description	Calories	Protein	Fat	Net Carbs	Serving Size
FRUITS	JUICE	LEMON JUICE, RAW	7	0	0	2	1 FL OZ
FRUITS	JUICE	LIME JUICE, CANNED OR BOTTLED, UNSWEETENED	6	0	0	2	1 FL OZ
FRUITS	JUICE	LIME JUICE, RAW	8	0	0	3	1 FL OZ
FRUITS	JUICE	ORANGE JUICE, CANNED, UNSWEETENED	15	0	0	3	1 FL OZ
FRUITS	JUICE	ORANGE JUICE, CHILLED, INCLUDES FROM CONCENTRATE	15	0	0	4	1 FL OZ
FRUITS	JUICE	ORANGE JUICE, FROZEN CONCENTRATE, UNSWEETENED, DILUTED WITH 3 VOLUME WATER	12	0	0	3	1 FL OZ
FRUITS	JUICE	ORANGE JUICE, RAW	14	0	0	3	1 FL OZ
FRUITS	JUICE	ORANGE-GRAPEFRUIT JUICE, CANNED OR BOTTLED, UNSWEETENED	13	0	0	3	1 FL OZ
FRUITS	JUICE	POMEGRANATE JUICE, BOTTLED	17	0	0	4	1 FL OZ
GRAINS	BREAD	BREAD, LOW CARB	60	6	2	1	1 SLICE, 1 OZ
GRAINS	BREAD	TORTILLAS, LOW CARB, WHITE, FLOUR	90	3	2	4	1 TORTILLA, 28G
GRAINS	BREAD	TORTILLAS, LOW CARB, WHOLE WHEAT, FLOUR	90	3	2	3	1 TORTILLA, 28G
GRAINS	CEREAL	CEREALS, CORN GRITS, WHITE, REGULAR AND QUICK	11	0	0	2	1 TBSP.
GRAINS	CEREAL	CEREALS, OATS, INSTANT, FORTIFIED, WITH CINNAMON AND SPICE, PREPARED WITH WATER	14	0	0	3	1 TBSP.
GRAINS	CEREAL GRAINS	BULGUR, COOKED	7	0	0	2	1 TBSP.
GRAINS	CEREAL GRAINS	CORN FLOUR, WHOLE-GRAIN, BLUE (HARINA DE MAIZ MORADO)	22	1	0	3	1 TBSP.
GRAINS	COOKIE	COOKIES, ANIMAL CRACKERS (INCLUDES ARROWROOT, TEA BISCUITS)	22	0	1	4	1 BISCUIT

FOODS WITH LESS THAN 5 CARBS AND NO MORE THAN 1

Food Group	Sub Group	Food Description	Calories	Protein	Fat	Net Carbs	Serving Size
GRAINS	COOKIE	COOKIES, BUTTER	23	0	1	3	1 COOKIE
GRAINS	COOKIE	COOKIES, VANILLA WAFERS, HIGHER FAT	28	0	1	4	1 COOKIE
GRAINS	CRACKER	CRACKERS, CHEESE, SANDWICH-TYPE WITH CHEESE FILLING	32	1	2	4	1 CRACKER, SANDWICH
GRAINS	CRACKER	CRACKERS, SALTINES, INCLUDES OYSTER, SODA, SOUP	13	0	0	2	1 CRACKER
GRAINS	CRACKER	CRACKERS, STANDARD SNACK-TYPE, SANDWICH, WITH CHEESE FILLING	33	1	1	4	1 CRACKER, SANDWICH
GRAINS	CRACKER	CRACKERS, STANDARD SNACK-TYPE, SANDWICH, WITH PEANUT BUTTER FILLING	35	1	2	4	1 CRACKER, SANDWICH
GRAINS	SNACKS	POPCORN, MICROWAVE, REGULAR (BUTTER) FLAVOR, MADE WITH PALM OIL	37	1	2	3	1 CUP
GRAINS	SNACKS	SNACKS, POPCORN, MICROWAVE, REGULAR (BUTTER) FLAVOR, MADE WITH PARTIALLY HYDROGENATED OIL	39	1	2	3	1 CUP
GRAINS	SNACKS	SNACKS, POPCORN, OIL-POPPED, MICROWAVE, REGULAR FLAVOR, NO TRANS FAT	64	1	5	4	1 CUP
OTHER	BEVERAGE	BEVERAGE, ENERGY DRINK, SUGAR FREE	10	1	0	1	8 FL OZ
OTHER	BEVERAGE	BEVERAGE, FORTIFIED LOW CALORIE FRUIT JUICE BEVERAGE	19	0	0	3	16.9 FL OZ
OTHER	BEVERAGE	COFFEE, INSTANT, REGULAR, POWDER	4	0	0	1	1 TSP
OTHER	BEVERAGE	COFFEE, INSTANT, WITH CHICORY, POWDER	4	0	0	1	1 TSP
OTHER	BEVERAGE	SAKE	39	0	0	1	1 FL OZ
OTHER	BEVERAGE	TEA, BLACK, BREWED	2	0	0	1	6 FL OZ
OTHER	BEVERAGE	TEA, INSTANT, SWEETENED WITH NON-NUTRITIVE SWEETENER	3	0	0	1	2 TSP

FOODS WITH LESS THAN 5 CARBS AND NO MORE THAN 1

Food Group	Sub Group	Food Description	Calories	Protein	Fat	Net Carbs	Serving Size
OTHER	BEVERAGE	VEGETABLE AND FRUIT JUICE DRINK, REDUCED CALORIE, WITH LOW-CALORIE SWEETENER, ADDED VITAMIN C	10	0	0	3	1 SERVING
OTHER	BEVERAGE	WINE, TABLE, RED	125	0	0	4	5 FL OZ
OTHER	BEVERAGE	WINE, TABLE, RED, CABERNET SAUVIGNON	122	0	0	4	5 FL OZ
OTHER	BEVERAGE	WINE, TABLE, RED, CLARET	122	0	0	4	5 FL OZ
OTHER	BEVERAGE	WINE, TABLE, RED, MERLOT	122	0	0	4	5 FL OZ
OTHER	BEVERAGE	WINE, TABLE, RED, PETITE SYRAH	125	0	0	4	5 FL OZ
OTHER	BEVERAGE	WINE, TABLE, RED, PINOT NOIR	121	0	0	3	5 FL OZ
OTHER	BEVERAGE	WINE, TABLE, RED, SYRAH	122	0	0	4	5 FL OZ
OTHER	BEVERAGE	WINE, TABLE, RED, ZINFANDEL	129	0	0	4	5 FL OZ
OTHER	BEVERAGE	WINE, TABLE, WHITE	121	0	0	4	5 FL OZ
OTHER	BEVERAGE	WINE, TABLE, WHITE, CHARDONNAY	123	0	0	3	5 FL OZ
OTHER	BEVERAGE	WINE, TABLE, WHITE, FUME BLANC	121	0	0	3	5 FL OZ
OTHER	BEVERAGE	WINE, TABLE, WHITE, GEWURZTRAMINER	119	0	0	4	5 FL OZ
OTHER	BEVERAGE	WINE, TABLE, WHITE, PINOT BLANC	119	0	0	3	5 FL OZ
OTHER	BEVERAGE	WINE, TABLE, WHITE, PINOT GRIS (GRIGIO)	122	0	0	3	5 FL OZ
OTHER	BEVERAGE	WINE, TABLE, WHITE, SAUVIGNON BLANC	119	0	0	3	5 FL OZ
OTHER	GRAVY	AU JUS GRAVY, CANNED	9	1	0	1	1/4 CUP
OTHER	GRAVY	BROWN GRAVY, INSTANT, DRY	23	1	1	4	1 SERVING
OTHER	GRAVY	TURKEY GRAVY, CANNED, READY-TO-SERVE	8	0	0	1	1 TBSP.
OTHER	SAUCE	ALFREDO CREAM SAUCE	228	6	26	2	2 OZ
OTHER	SAUCE	CHEESE SAUCE, READY-TO-SERVE	110	4	8	4	1/4 CUP

FOODS WITH LESS THAN 5 CARBS AND NO MORE THAN 1

Food Group	Sub Group	Food Description	Calories	Protein	Fat	Net Carbs	Serving Size
OTHER	SAUCE	CHILI, PEPPERS, HOT, IMMATURE GREEN SAUCE, CANNED	3	0	0	1	1 TBSP.
OTHER	SAUCE	DIP, GUACAMOLE	240	4	20	4	1/2 CUP
OTHER	SAUCE	FISH SAUCE, READY-TO-SERVE	6	1	0	1	1 TBSP.
OTHER	SAUCE	OYSTER SAUCE, READY-TO-SERVE	9	0	0	2	1 TBSP.
OTHER	SAUCE	PASTA SAUCE, MARINARA, READY-TO-SERVE	80	1	7	3	1/2 CUP
OTHER	SAUCE	PEPPERS, HOT, CHILI, MATURE RED, CANNED SAUCE	3	0	0	1	1 TBSP.
OTHER	SAUCE	PIZZA SAUCE, CANNED, READY-TO-SERVE	34	1	1	4	1/4 CUP
OTHER	SAUCE	SALSA SAUCE, VERDE, READY-TO-SERVE	11	0	0	1	2 TBSP.
OTHER	SAUCE	TARTAR SAUCE, READY-TO-SERVE	63	0	5	4	2 TBSP.
OTHER	SAUCE	TERIYAKI SAUCE, READY-TO-SERVE	16	1	0	3	1 TBSP.
OTHER	SAUCE	TOMATO CHILI BOTTLED SAUCE	6	0	0	1	1 PACKET
OTHER	SAUCE	WING HOT SAUCE, READY-TO-SERVE	30	0	3	1	1 TBSP.
OTHER	SAUCE	WORCESTERSHIRE SAUCE	13	0	0	3	1 TBSP.
OTHER	SNACKS	SNACKS, BEEF JERKY, CHOPPED AND FORMED	115	9	7	2	1 OZ
OTHER	SOUP	CHICKEN BROTH, CANNED SOUP, CONDENSED	39	6	1	1	1/2 CUP
OTHER	SOUP	CHICKEN BROTH, READY-TO-SERVE	15	2	1	1	1 CUP
OTHER	SOUP	CHILI BEEF, CANNED SOUP, PREPARED WITH EQUAL VOLUME WATER	19	1	0	3	1 FL OZ
OTHER	SOUP	FISH BROTH	39	5	1	1	1 CUP
OTHER	SOUP	RAMEN NOODLE SOUP, ANY FLAVOR, DRY	26	1	1	3	1 PACKET
OTHER	SOUP	TOMATO, CANNED SOUP, PREPARED WITH WATER	9	0	0	2	1 FL OZ

FOODS WITH LESS THAN 5 CARBS AND NO MORE THAN 1

Food Group	Sub Group	Food Description	Calories	Protein	Fat	Net Carbs	Serving Size
OTHER	SPICES AND HERBS	BALSAMIC VINEGAR	14	0	0	3	1 TBSP.
OTHER	SPICES AND HERBS	HORSERADISH, PREPARED	7	0	0	2	1 TBSP.
OTHER	SPICES AND HERBS	ONION POWDER	24	1	0	4	1 TBSP.
OTHER	SPICES AND HERBS	PEPPER, BLACK	17	1	0	2	1 TBSP.
OTHER	SPICES AND HERBS	PEPPER, RED OR CAYENNE	17	1	1	2	1 TBSP.
OTHER	SPICES AND HERBS	PEPPER, WHITE	21	1	0	3	1 TBSP.
OTHER	SWEETS	BAKING CHOCOLATE, UNSWEETENED, SQUARES	186	4	15	3	1 OZ, SQUARE BAKERS
OTHER	SWEETS	CANDIES, GUM DROPS, DIETETIC OR LOW CALORIE (SORBITOL)	8	0	0	3	1 PIECE
OTHER	SWEETS	CANDIES, HARD, DIETETIC OR LOW CALORIE (SORBITOL)	12	0	0	3	1 PIECE
OTHER	SWEETS	CANDIES, MILK CHOCOLATE	37	1	2	4	1 MINIATURE BAR
OTHER	SWEETS	CHEWING GUM	11	0	0	3	1 STICK
OTHER	SWEETS	CHEWING GUM, SUGARLESS	5	0	0	2	1 PIECE
OTHER	SWEETS	COCOA, DRY POWDER, UNSWEETENED	12	1	1	1	1 TBSP.
OTHER	SWEETS	FROZEN NOVELTIES, ICE TYPE, FRUIT, NO SUGAR ADDED	12	0	0	3	1 BAR
OTHER	SWEETS	FROZEN NOVELTIES, ICE TYPE, POP, WITH LOW CALORIE SWEETENER	13	0	0	3	1.75 FL OZ POP
OTHER	SWEETS	SWEETENER, HERBAL EXTRACT POWDER FROM STEVIA LEAF	0	0	0	1	1 PACKAGE
OTHER	SWEETS	SWEETENERS, TABLETOP, ASPARTAME, EQUAL, PACKETS	11	0	0	3	1 TSP
OTHER	SWEETS	SWEETENERS, TABLETOP, SACCHARIN (SODIUM SACCHARIN)	3	0	0	1	1 PACKET

FOODS WITH LESS THAN 5 CARBS AND NO MORE THAN 1

Food Group	Sub Group	Food Description	Calories	Protein	Fat	Net Carbs	Serving Size
OTHER	SWEETS	SWEETENERS, TABLETOP, SUCRALOSE, SPLENDA PACKETS	3	0	0	1	1 PACKET
PROTEIN	BEEF	BEEF, TOP LOIN PETITE ROAST	194	23	11	1	3 OZ
PROTEIN	CHICKEN	CHICKEN, CANNED, NO BROTH	379	52	17	2	1 CUP
PROTEIN	CHICKEN	CHICKEN, ROASTING, GIBLETS, SIMMERED	239	39	8	1	1 CUP
PROTEIN	EGG	EGG SUBSTITUTE, POWDER	40	5	1	2	1/3 OZ
PROTEIN	EGG	EGG, WHOLE, COOKED, HARD-BOILED	211	17	14	2	1 CUP
PROTEIN	LEGUME	CHILI WITH BEANS, CANNED	18	1	1	1	1 TBSP.
PROTEIN	LEGUME	HUMMUS	25	1	1	1	1 TBSP.
PROTEIN	LEGUME	KIDNEY BEANS, RED, MATURE SEEDS, CANNED, SOLIDS AND LIQUIDS	13	1	0	1	1 TBSP.
PROTEIN	LEGUME	LENTILS, MATURE SEEDS, COOKED, BOILED	14	1	0	1	1 TBSP.
PROTEIN	LEGUME	LIMA BEANS, LARGE, MATURE SEEDS, COOKED, BOILED	13	1	0	1	1 TBSP.
PROTEIN	LEGUME	MISO	34	2	1	3	1 TBSP.
PROTEIN	LEGUME	PEANUT BUTTER WITH OMEGA-3, CREAMY	97	4	9	2	1 TBSP.
PROTEIN	LEGUME	PEANUT BUTTER, CHUNK STYLE	188	8	16	4	2 TBSP.
PROTEIN	LEGUME	PEANUTS, ALL TYPES, DRY-ROASTED	166	7	14	4	1 OZ
PROTEIN	LEGUME	PEANUTS, VIRGINIA, OIL-ROASTED	164	7	14	3	1 OZ
PROTEIN	LEGUME	PEAS, SPLIT, MATURE SEEDS, COOKED, BOILED	14	1	0	2	1 TBSP.
PROTEIN	LEGUME	PINTO BEANS, MATURE SEEDS, COOKED, BOILED	15	1	0	2	1 TBSP.
PROTEIN	LEGUME	REFRIED BEANS, CANNED, TRADITIONAL, REDUCED SODIUM	14	1	0	1	1 TBSP.
PROTEIN	LEGUME	SOY SAUCE MADE FROM HYDROLYZED VEGETABLE PROTEIN	11	1	0	1	1 TBSP.

FOODS WITH LESS THAN 5 CARBS AND NO MORE THAN 1

Food Group	Sub Group	Food Description	Calories	Protein	Fat	Net Carbs	Serving Size
PROTEIN	LEGUME	SOY SAUCE MADE FROM SOY (TAMARI)	11	2	0	1	1 TBSP.
PROTEIN	LEGUME	SOY SAUCE MADE FROM SOY AND WHEAT (SHOYU)	8	1	0	1	1 TBSP.
PROTEIN	LEGUME	SOY SAUCE, REDUCED SODIUM, MADE FROM HYDROLYZED VEGETABLE PROTEIN	14	1	0	2	1 TBSP.
PROTEIN	LEGUME	TEMPEH	173	17	6	3	3 OZ
PROTEIN	LEGUME	TOFU, EXTRA FIRM, PREPARED WITH NIGARI	83	9	5	2	1 BLOCK
PROTEIN	LEGUME	TOFU, FIRM, PREPARED WITH CALCIUM SULFATE AND MAGNESIUM CHLORIDE (NIGARI)	88	10	5	1	1/2 CUP
PROTEIN	LEGUME	TOFU, FRIED	76	5	6	2	1 OZ
PROTEIN	LEGUME	TOFU, HARD, PREPARED WITH NIGARI	178	15	12	4	1 BLOCK
PROTEIN	LEGUME	TOFU, SOFT, PREPARED WITH CALCIUM SULFATE AND MAGNESIUM CHLORIDE (NIGARI)	151	16	9	4	1 CUP
PROTEIN	LEGUME	VEGETARIAN FILLETS	247	20	15	3	1 FILLET
PROTEIN	LEGUME	VEGETARIAN MEATLOAF OR PATTIES	110	12	5	1	1 SLICE
PROTEIN	LUNCH MEAT	BEEF, DRIED	43	9	1	1	10 SLICES
PROTEIN	LUNCH MEAT	BOLOGNA, MEAT AND POULTRY	93	3	8	2	1 SLICE
PROTEIN	LUNCH MEAT	BRATWURST, BEEF AND PORK, SMOKED	196	8	17	1	2 1/3 OZ
PROTEIN	LUNCH MEAT	BRAUNSCHWEIGER (A LIVER SAUSAGE), PORK	92	4	8	1	1 OZ
PROTEIN	LUNCH MEAT	CHORIZO, PORK AND BEEF	127	7	11	1	1 OZ
PROTEIN	LUNCH MEAT	FRANKFURTER, BEEF AND PORK	137	5	12	1	1 FRANK-FURTER
PROTEIN	LUNCH MEAT	FRANKFURTER, CHICKEN	100	7	7	1	1 FRANK-FURTER

FOODS WITH LESS THAN 5 CARBS AND NO MORE THAN 1

Food Group	Sub Group	Food Description	Calories	Protein	Fat	Net Carbs	Serving Size
PROTEIN	LUNCH MEAT	FRANKFURTER, TURKEY	100	6	8	2	1 FRANK-FURTER
PROTEIN	LUNCH MEAT	HAM AND CHEESE LOAF OR ROLL	67	4	5	1	1 SLICE, 4" × 4" × 3/32" THICK
PROTEIN	LUNCH MEAT	HAM, CHOPPED, NOT CANNED	50	5	3	1	1 SLICE, 4" × 4" × 3/32" THICK
PROTEIN	LUNCH MEAT	HAM, HONEY, SMOKED, COOKED	67	10	1	4	1.94 OZ
PROTEIN	LUNCH MEAT	HAM, SLICED, REGULAR	46	5	2	1	1 SLICE
PROTEIN	LUNCH MEAT	KIELBASA, FULLY GRILLED	286	11	25	4	3 OZ
PROTEIN	LUNCH MEAT	KIELBASA, POLISH, TURKEY AND BEEF, SMOKED	127	7	10	2	2 OZ
PROTEIN	LUNCH MEAT	KNACKWURST, KNOCKWURST, PORK, BEEF	87	3	8	1	1 OZ
PROTEIN	LUNCH MEAT	LIVERWURST SPREAD	168	7	14	2	1/4 CUP
PROTEIN	LUNCH MEAT	OLIVE LOAF, PORK	66	3	5	3	1 SLICE, 4" × 4" × 3/32" THICK
PROTEIN	LUNCH MEAT	OVEN-ROASTED CHICKEN BREAST ROLL	75	8	4	1	2 OZ
PROTEIN	LUNCH MEAT	PASTRAMI, TURKEY	79	9	4	2	2 SLICES
PROTEIN	LUNCH MEAT	SALAMI, BEEF	74	4	6	1	1 OZ
PROTEIN	LUNCH MEAT	TURKEY BREAST, LUNCH MEAT	32	6	0	1	1 SLICE
PROTEIN	LUNCH MEAT	TURKEY BREAST, SLICED, OVEN ROASTED, LUNCH MEAT	22	4	0	1	1 SLICE
PROTEIN	LUNCH MEAT	TURKEY, WHITE, ROTISSERIE, DELI CUT	54	6	1	4	1.69 OZ
PROTEIN	MEAT SUBSTITUTE	BACON BITS, MEATLESS	33	2	2	1	1 TBSP.
PROTEIN	MEAT SUBSTITUTE	FISH STICKS, MEATLESS	81	6	5	1	1 STICK
PROTEIN	MEAT SUBSTITUTE	LUNCHEON SLICES, MEATLESS	26	2	2	1	1 SLICE

FOODS WITH LESS THAN 5 CARBS AND NO MORE THAN 1

Food Group	Sub Group	Food Description	Calories	Protein	Fat	Net Carbs	Serving Size
PROTEIN	MEAT SUBSTITUTE	SANDWICH SPREAD, MEATLESS	22	1	1	1	1 TBSP.
PROTEIN	MEAT SUBSTITUTE	SAUSAGE, MEATLESS	64	5	5	1	1 LINK
PROTEIN	MEAT SUBSTITUTE	VEGETARIAN FILLETS	247	20	15	3	1 FILLET
PROTEIN	MEAT SUBSTITUTE	VEGETARIAN MEATLOAF OR PATTIES	110	12	5	1	1 SLICE
PROTEIN	NUT	ALMOND BUTTER, PLAIN	98	3	9	1	1 TBSP.
PROTEIN	NUT	CASHEW BUTTER, PLAIN	94	3	8	4	1 TBSP.
PROTEIN	NUT	COCONUT BUTTER, PLAIN	190	2	18	2	2 TBSP.
PROTEIN	NUT	COCONUT CREAM, RAW (LIQUID EXPRESSED FROM GRATED MEAT)	50	1	5	1	1 TBSP.
PROTEIN	NUT	COCONUT MEAT, DRIED (DESICCATED), NOT SWEETENED	185	2	18	2	1 OZ
PROTEIN	NUT	PECANS, DRY ROASTED	199	3	21	1	1 OZ
PROTEIN	NUT	PECANS, OIL ROASTED	787	10	83	4	1 CUP
PROTEIN	NUT	WALNUTS, BLACK, DRIED	774	30	74	3	1 CUP
PROTEIN	PORK	HAM – WATER ADDED, RUMP, BONE-IN, ROASTED	137	17	7	1	3 OZ
PROTEIN	PORK	HAM – WATER ADDED, SHANK, BONE-IN, ROASTED	170	16	11	1	3 OZ
PROTEIN	PORK	HAM – WATER ADDED, SLICE, BONE-IN, PAN-BROIL	141	18	7	1	3 OZ
PROTEIN	PORK	HAM – WATER ADDED, SLICE, PAN-BROIL	106	16	4	1	3 OZ
PROTEIN	PORK	HAM AND WATER PRODUCT, RUMP, BONE-IN, ROASTED	158	17	10	1	3 OZ
PROTEIN	PORK	HAM AND WATER PRODUCT, SHANK, BONE-IN, ROASTED	199	15	15	1	3 OZ
PROTEIN	PORK	HAM AND WATER PRODUCT, SLICE, BONE-IN, PAN-BROIL	132	17	7	1	3 OZ
PROTEIN	PORK	HAM AND WATER PRODUCT, SLICE, PAN-BROIL	105	13	4	4	3 OZ

FOODS WITH LESS THAN 5 CARBS AND NO MORE THAN 1

Food Group	Sub Group	Food Description	Calories	Protein	Fat	Net Carbs	Serving Size
PROTEIN	PORK	HAM AND WATER PRODUCT, WHOLE, ROASTED	105	12	5	4	3 OZ
PROTEIN	PORK	HAM, RUMP, BONE-IN, ROASTED	150	20	8	1	3 OZ
PROTEIN	PORK	HAM, SHANK, BONE-IN, ROASTED	162	21	8	1	3 OZ
PROTEIN	PORK	HAM, SLICE, BONE-IN, PAN-BROIL	153	22	7	1	3 OZ
PROTEIN	PORK	PORK, BLADE (CHOPS)	265	32	15	1	1 CHOP
PROTEIN	PORK	PORK, GROUND, 72% LEAN / 28% FAT	444	26	37	2	4 OZ
PROTEIN	SAUSAGE	POLISH SAUSAGE, PORK	277	12	24	1	3 OZ
PROTEIN	SAUSAGE	SAUSAGE, ITALIAN, PORK, COOKED	286	16	23	4	1 LINK, 4/LB.
PROTEIN	SAUSAGE	SAUSAGE, ITALIAN, SWEET, LINKS	125	14	7	2	1 LINK, 3 OZ
PROTEIN	SAUSAGE	SAUSAGE, POLISH, PORK AND BEEF, SMOKED	229	9	20	2	2.67 OZ
PROTEIN	SAUSAGE	SAUSAGE, SMOKED LINK SAUSAGE, PORK AND BEEF	272	10	24	2	3 OZ
PROTEIN	SAUSAGE	SAUSAGE, SUMMER, PORK AND BEEF, STICKS, WITH CHEDDAR CHEESE	119	5	11	1	1 OZ
PROTEIN	SAUSAGE	SAUSAGE, TURKEY, BREAKFAST LINKS, MILD	132	9	10	1	2 OZ, 2 LINKS
PROTEIN	SAUSAGE	SAUSAGE, TURKEY, HOT, SMOKED	88	8	5	2	2 OZ
PROTEIN	SAUSAGE	SMOKED LINK SAUSAGE, PORK	210	8	19	1	1 LINK, (4" LONG × 1-1/8" DIA)
PROTEIN	SEAFOOD	CLAM, MIXED SPECIES	126	22	2	4	3 OZ
PROTEIN	SEED	SESAME BUTTER, PASTE	94	3	8	3	1 TBSP.
PROTEIN	SEED	SESAME BUTTER, TAHINI, FROM ROASTED AND TOASTED KERNELS (MOST COMMON TYPE)	89	3	8	2	1 TBSP.
PROTEIN	SEED	SESAME BUTTER, TAHINI, TYPE OF KERNELS UNSPECIFIED	89	3	8	2	1 TBSP.

FOODS WITH LESS THAN 5 CARBS AND NO MORE THAN 1

Food Group	Sub Group	Food Description	Calories	Protein	Fat	Net Carbs	Serving Size
PROTEIN	SEED	SESAME SEEDS, WHOLE, ROASTED AND TOASTED	158	5	13	3	1 OZ
PROTEIN	SEED	SUNFLOWER SEED BUTTER	99	3	9	3	1 TBSP.
PROTEIN	SEED	SUNFLOWER SEED KERNELS FROM SHELL, DRY ROASTED	155	5	14	1	1 OZ
PROTEIN	SEED	SUNFLOWER SEED KERNELS, OIL ROASTED	168	6	15	3	1 OZ
PROTEIN	SHELLFISH	CRAB, DUNGENESS	94	19	1	1	3 OZ
PROTEIN	SHELLFISH	SHRIMP, MIXED SPECIES	101	19	1	1	3 OZ
PROTEIN	TURKEY	TURKEY ROAST, FROZEN, SEASONED, LIGHT AND DARK MEAT, ROASTED	209	29	8	4	1 CUP
VEGETABLE	VEGETABLE	ARTICHOKES (GLOBE OR FRENCH), COOKED	64	3	0	4	1 ARTICHOKE, MEDIUM
VEGETABLE	VEGETABLE	ASPARAGUS, CANNED, SOLIDS AND LIQUIDS	18	2	0	2	1/2 CUP
VEGETABLE	VEGETABLE	ASPARAGUS, RAW	27	3	0	2	1 CUP
VEGETABLE	VEGETABLE	BAMBOO SHOOTS, CANNED, DRAINED SOLIDS	25	2	1	2	1 CUP
VEGETABLE	VEGETABLE	BEANS, MUNG, MATURE SEEDS, SPROUTED, CANNED, DRAINED SOLIDS	15	2	0	2	1 CUP
VEGETABLE	VEGETABLE	BEANS, SNAP, GREEN, RAW	31	2	0	4	1 CUP
VEGETABLE	VEGETABLE	BEANS, SNAP, YELLOW, RAW	31	2	0	4	1 CUP
VEGETABLE	VEGETABLE	BEET GREENS, COOKED	39	4	0	4	1 CUP
VEGETABLE	VEGETABLE	BEET GREENS, RAW	8	1	0	1	1 CUP
VEGETABLE	VEGETABLE	BROCCOLI RAAB, COOKED	28	3	0	1	1 SERVING
VEGETABLE	VEGETABLE	BROCCOLI, CHINESE, COOKED	19	1	1	1	1 CUP
VEGETABLE	VEGETABLE	BROCCOLI, CHOPPED, COOKED	52	6	0	4	1 CUP
VEGETABLE	VEGETABLE	BROCCOLI, COOKED	27	2	0	3	1/2 CUP
VEGETABLE	VEGETABLE	BROCCOLI, FLOWER CLUSTERS, RAW	20	2	0	3	1 CUP

FOODS WITH LESS THAN 5 CARBS AND NO MORE THAN 1

Food Group	Sub Group	Food Description	Calories	Protein	Fat	Net Carbs	Serving Size
VEGETABLE	VEGETABLE	BROCCOLI, RAW	31	3	0	4	1 CUP
VEGETABLE	VEGETABLE	CABBAGE, COMMON, COOKED	17	1	0	3	1/2 CUP
VEGETABLE	VEGETABLE	CABBAGE, COMMON, RAW	8	0	0	1	1/2 CUP
VEGETABLE	VEGETABLE	CABBAGE, RED, COOKED	22	1	0	3	1/2 CUP
VEGETABLE	VEGETABLE	CABBAGE, RED, RAW	22	1	0	4	1 CUP
VEGETABLE	VEGETABLE	CARROTS, BABY, RAW	4	0	0	1	1 MEDIUM
VEGETABLE	VEGETABLE	CARROTS, COOKED	27	1	0	4	1/2 CUP
VEGETABLE	VEGETABLE	CAULIFLOWER, COOKED	31	3	0	1	1 CUP
VEGETABLE	VEGETABLE	CAULIFLOWER, RAW	27	2	0	3	1 CUP
VEGETABLE	VEGETABLE	CELERY, COOKED	27	1	0	4	1 CUP
VEGETABLE	VEGETABLE	CELERY, RAW	16	1	0	1	1 CUP
VEGETABLE	VEGETABLE	CHARD, SWISS, COOKED	35	3	0	3	1 CUP
VEGETABLE	VEGETABLE	COLLARDS, COOKED	63	5	1	3	1 CUP
VEGETABLE	VEGETABLE	COLLARDS, RAW	12	1	0	1	1 CUP
VEGETABLE	VEGETABLE	CRESS, GARDEN, COOKED	31	3	1	4	1 CUP
VEGETABLE	VEGETABLE	CRESS, GARDEN, RAW	16	1	0	2	1 CUP
VEGETABLE	VEGETABLE	CUCUMBER, PEELED, RAW	16	1	0	2	1 CUP
VEGETABLE	VEGETABLE	CUCUMBER, WITH PEEL, RAW	8	0	0	2	1/2 CUP
VEGETABLE	VEGETABLE	EGGPLANT, RAW	21	1	0	3	1 CUP
VEGETABLE	VEGETABLE	FENNEL, BULB, RAW	27	1	0	3	1 CUP
VEGETABLE	VEGETABLE	GARLIC, RAW	4	0	0	1	1 TSP
VEGETABLE	VEGETABLE	HEARTS OF PALM, CANNED	41	4	1	3	1 CUP
VEGETABLE	VEGETABLE	KALE, COOKED	36	2	1	4	1 CUP
VEGETABLE	VEGETABLE	KOHLRABI, RAW	36	2	0	3	1 CUP
VEGETABLE	VEGETABLE	LEEKS (BULB AND LOWER LEAF-PORTION), COOKED	8	0	0	2	1/4 CUP

FOODS WITH LESS THAN 5 CARBS AND NO MORE THAN 1

Food Group	Sub Group	Food Description	Calories	Protein	Fat	Net Carbs	Serving Size
VEGETABLE	VEGETABLE	LETTUCE, COS OR ROMAINE, RAW	8	1	0	1	1 CUP
VEGETABLE	VEGETABLE	LETTUCE, GREEN LEAF, RAW	5	0	0	1	1 CUP
VEGETABLE	VEGETABLE	LETTUCE, ICEBERG (INCLUDES CRISP HEAD TYPES), RAW	10	1	0	1	1 CUP
VEGETABLE	VEGETABLE	LETTUCE, RED LEAF, RAW	4	0	0	1	1 CUP
VEGETABLE	VEGETABLE	MUSHROOMS, BROWN, ITALIAN, OR CRIMINI, RAW	19	2	0	3	1 CUP
VEGETABLE	VEGETABLE	MUSHROOMS, CANNED, DRAINED SOLIDS	39	3	0	4	1 CUP
VEGETABLE	VEGETABLE	MUSHROOMS, MAITAKE, RAW	22	1	0	3	1 CUP
VEGETABLE	VEGETABLE	MUSHROOMS, OYSTER, RAW	5	0	0	1	1 SMALL
VEGETABLE	VEGETABLE	MUSHROOMS, PORTABELLA, GRILLED	35	4	1	2	1 CUP
VEGETABLE	VEGETABLE	MUSHROOMS, PORTABELLA, RAW	19	2	0	2	1 CUP
VEGETABLE	VEGETABLE	MUSHROOMS, SHIITAKE, RAW	6	0	0	1	1 PIECE, WHOLE
VEGETABLE	VEGETABLE	MUSHROOMS, SHIITAKE, STIR-FRIED	38	3	0	4	1 CUP
VEGETABLE	VEGETABLE	MUSHROOMS, WHITE, RAW	21	3	0	2	1 CUP
VEGETABLE	VEGETABLE	MUSTARD GREENS, COOKED	36	4	1	3	1 CUP
VEGETABLE	VEGETABLE	MUSTARD GREENS, RAW	15	2	0	1	1 CUP
VEGETABLE	VEGETABLE	OKRA, COOKED	27	1	0	4	1/2 CUP
VEGETABLE	VEGETABLE	OKRA, RAW	33	2	0	4	1 CUP
VEGETABLE	VEGETABLE	ONIONS, COOKED	7	0	0	2	1 TBSP.
VEGETABLE	VEGETABLE	ONIONS, DEHYDRATED FLAKES	17	0	0	4	1 TBSP.
VEGETABLE	VEGETABLE	ONIONS, SPRING OR SCALLIONS (INCLUDES TOPS AND BULB), RAW	32	2	0	4	1 CUP
VEGETABLE	VEGETABLE	PARSLEY, FRESH	22	2	0	2	1 CUP

FOODS WITH LESS THAN 5 CARBS AND NO MORE THAN 1

Food Group	Sub Group	Food Description	Calories	Protein	Fat	Net Carbs	Serving Size
VEGETABLE	VEGETABLE	PEAS, EDIBLE-PODDED, RAW	41	3	0	4	1 CUP
VEGETABLE	VEGETABLE	PEPPERS, CHILI, GREEN, CANNED	29	1	0	4	1 CUP
VEGETABLE	VEGETABLE	PEPPERS, HOT CHILI, RED, CANNED, EXCLUDING SEEDS, SOLIDS AND LIQUIDS	14	1	0	2	1/2 CUP
VEGETABLE	VEGETABLE	PEPPERS, JALAPENO, CANNED, SOLIDS AND LIQUIDS	37	1	1	2	1 CUP
VEGETABLE	VEGETABLE	PEPPERS, JALAPENO, RAW	26	1	0	3	1 CUP
VEGETABLE	VEGETABLE	PEPPERS, SWEET, GREEN, CANNED, SOLIDS AND LIQUIDS	25	1	0	3	1 CUP
VEGETABLE	VEGETABLE	PEPPERS, SWEET, GREEN, RAW	30	1	0	4	1 CUP
VEGETABLE	VEGETABLE	PICKLE RELISH, HOT DOG	14	0	0	4	1 TBSP.
VEGETABLE	VEGETABLE	PICKLES, CUCUMBER, SOUR	17	1	0	2	1 CUP
VEGETABLE	VEGETABLE	POTATOES, RAW, SKIN	22	1	0	4	1 SKIN
VEGETABLE	VEGETABLE	RADICCHIO, RAW	9	1	0	2	1 CUP
VEGETABLE	VEGETABLE	RADISHES, RAW	19	1	0	2	1 CUP
VEGETABLE	VEGETABLE	SAUERKRAUT, CANNED, SOLIDS AND LIQUIDS	45	2	0	3	1 CUP
VEGETABLE	VEGETABLE	SEAWEED	5	0	0	1	2 TBSP.
VEGETABLE	VEGETABLE	SHALLOTS, RAW	7	0	0	2	1 TBSP.
VEGETABLE	VEGETABLE	SPINACH, CANNED, SOLIDS AND LIQUIDS	44	5	1	2	1 CUP
VEGETABLE	VEGETABLE	SPINACH, COOKED, BOILED	41	5	0	3	1 CUP
VEGETABLE	VEGETABLE	SPINACH, FROZEN, CHOPPED OR LEAF, COOKED, BOILED	32	4	1	1	1/2 CUP
VEGETABLE	VEGETABLE	SQUASH, SUMMER, ALL VARIETIES, RAW	18	1	0	3	1 CUP
VEGETABLE	VEGETABLE	TOMATILLOS, RAW	21	1	1	3	1/2 CUP

FOODS WITH LESS THAN 5 CARBS AND NO MORE THAN 1

Food Group	Sub Group	Food Description	Calories	Protein	Fat	Net Carbs	Serving Size
VEGETABLE	VEGETABLE	TOMATOES, RED CHERRY, RAW	27	1	0	4	1 CUP
VEGETABLE	VEGETABLE	TOMATOES, SUN-DRIED, PACKED IN OIL, DRAINED	6	0	0	1	1 PIECE
VEGETABLE	VEGETABLE	TOMATOES, YELLOW, RAW	21	1	0	3	1 CUP
VEGETABLE	VEGETABLE	TURNIP GREENS, RAW	18	1	0	2	1 CUP
VEGETABLE	VEGETABLE JUICE	TOMATO AND VEGETABLE JUICE, LOW SODIUM	7	0	0	1	1 FL OZ
VEGETABLE	VEGETABLE JUICE	TOMATO JUICE, CANNED	5	0	0	1	1 FL OZ

FOODS WITH 0 CARBS

Food Group	Sub-Group	Food Description	Calories	Protein	Fat	Net Carbs	Serving Size
DAIRY	BUTTER	BUTTER, SALTED	102	0	12	0	1 TBSP.
DAIRY	BUTTER	BUTTER, WHIPPED	67	0	8	0	1 TBSP.
DAIRY	CHEESE	CHEESE, BRIE	94	6	8	0	1 OZ
DAIRY	CHEESE	CHEESE, CAMEMBERT	84	6	7	0	1 OZ
DAIRY	CHEESE	CHEESE, EDAM	100	7	8	0	1 OZ
DAIRY	CHEESE	CHEESE, GOAT, SEMISOFT TYPE	102	6	8	0	1 OZ
DAIRY	CHEESE	CHEESE, GOAT, SOFT TYPE	74	5	6	0	1 OZ
DAIRY	CHEESE	CHEESE, GRUYERE	116	8	9	0	1 OZ
DAIRY	CHEESE	CHEESE, PARMESAN, SHREDDED	21	2	1	0	1 TBSP.
FATS & OILS	DRESSING	MAYONNAISE DRESSING	103	0	12	0	1 TBSP.
FATS & OILS	DRESSING	MAYONNAISE, MADE WITH TOFU	48	1	5	0	1 TBSP.
FATS & OILS	DRESSING	SALAD DRESSING, BACON AND TOMATO	49	0	5	0	1 TBSP.
FATS & OILS	DRESSING	SALAD DRESSING, CAESAR DRESSING	76	0	8	0	1 TBSP.

FOODS WITH 0 CARBS

Food Group	Sub-Group	Food Description	Calories	Protein	Fat	Net Carbs	Serving Size
FATS & OILS	DRESSING	SALAD DRESSING, MAYONNAISE	88	0	10	0	1 TBSP.
FATS & OILS	DRESSING	SALAD DRESSING, MAYONNAISE, SOYBEAN OIL	93	0	10	0	1 TBSP.
FATS & OILS	DRESSING	SALAD DRESSING, PEPPERCORN DRESSING	73	0	8	0	1 TBSP.
FATS & OILS	OIL	OIL, ALMOND	115	0	13	0	1 TBSP.
FATS & OILS	OIL	OIL, AVOCADO	124	0	14	0	1 TBSP.
FATS & OILS	OIL	OIL, CANOLA	124	0	14	0	1 TBSP.
FATS & OILS	OIL	OIL, COCONUT	112	0	13	0	1 TBSP.
FATS & OILS	OIL	OIL, CORN AND CANOLA	124	0	14	0	1 TBSP.
FATS & OILS	OIL	OIL, CORN, PEANUT, AND OLIVE	124	0	14	0	1 TBSP.
FATS & OILS	OIL	OIL, COTTONSEED, SALAD OR COOKING	115	0	13	0	1 TBSP.
FATS & OILS	OIL	OIL, FLAXSEED, COLD PRESSED	115	0	13	0	1 TBSP.
FATS & OILS	OIL	OIL, GRAPESEED	115	0	13	0	1 TBSP.
FATS & OILS	OIL	OIL, HAZELNUT	115	0	13	0	1 TBSP.
FATS & OILS	OIL	OIL, OLIVE, SALAD OR COOKING	115	0	13	0	1 TBSP.
FATS & OILS	OIL	OIL, PEANUT, SALAD OR COOKING	115	0	13	0	1 TBSP.
FATS & OILS	OIL	OIL, SAFFLOWER, SALAD OR COOKING	115	0	13	0	1 TBSP.
FATS & OILS	OIL	OIL, SESAME, SALAD OR COOKING	115	0	13	0	1 TBSP.
FATS & OILS	OIL	OIL, SUNFLOWER	115	0	13	0	1 TBSP.
FATS & OILS	OIL	OIL, SUNFLOWER, HIGH OLEIC (70% AND OVER)	124	0	14	0	1 TBSP.
FATS & OILS	OIL	OIL, WALNUT	115	0	13	0	1 TBSP.
FRUITS	FRUIT	LEMON PEEL, RAW	3	0	0	0	1 TBSP.
FRUITS	FRUIT	OLIVES, PICKLED, CANNED OR BOTTLED, GREEN	3	0	0	0	1 OLIVE

FOODS WITH 0 CARBS

Food Group	Sub-Group	Food Description	Calories	Protein	Fat	Net Carbs	Serving Size
FRUITS	FRUIT	OLIVES, RIPE, CANNED JUMBO	7	0	1	0	1 JUMBO
FRUITS	FRUIT	OLIVES, RIPE, CANNED LARGE	5	0	0	0	1 LARGE
OTHER	BEVERAGE	CARBONATED BEVERAGE, LOW CALORIE, COLA OR PEPPER-TYPES	0	0	0	0	1 CAN, (12 FL OZ)
OTHER	BEVERAGE	CARBONATED BEVERAGE, LOW CALORIE, OTHER THAN COLA OR PEPPER	0	0	0	0	1 CAN, (12 FL OZ)
OTHER	BEVERAGE	COFFEE, BREWED FROM GROUNDS, PREPARED WITH TAP WATER	0	0	0	0	6 FL OZ
OTHER	BEVERAGE	DISTILLED, GIN, 90 PROOF	110	0	0	0	1 JIGGER, FL OZ
OTHER	BEVERAGE	DISTILLED, RUM, 80 PROOF	97	0	0	0	1 JIGGER, FL OZ
OTHER	BEVERAGE	DISTILLED, VODKA, 80 PROOF	97	0	0	0	1 JIGGER, FL OZ
OTHER	BEVERAGE	DISTILLED, WHISKEY, 86 PROOF	105	0	0	0	1 JIGGER, FL OZ
OTHER	BEVERAGE	HIBISCUS TEA	0	0	0	0	8 FL OZ
OTHER	BEVERAGE	TEA, HERB, OTHER THAN CHAMOMILE, BREWED	2	0	0	0	6 FL OZ
OTHER	BEVERAGE	TEA, INSTANT, UNSWEETENED	0	0	0	0	1 TSP
OTHER	SAUCE	MUSTARD, YELLOW, PREPARED	6	0	0	0	2 TSP
OTHER	SAUCE	READY-TO-SERVE, PEPPER OR HOT SAUCE	0	0	0	0	1 TSP
OTHER	SAUCE	SRIRACHA SAUCE, READY-TO-SERVE	30	0	0	0	2 TBSP.
OTHER	SNACKS	SNACKS, PORK SKINS, BARBECUE-FLAVOR	151	16	9	0	1 OZ
OTHER	SNACKS	SNACKS, PORK SKINS, PLAIN	152	17	9	0	1 OZ
OTHER	SOUP	BEEF BROTH BOUILLON AND CONSOMMÉ, CANNED SOUP, CONDENSED	14	3	0	0	1/2 CUP
OTHER	SOUP	BEEF BROTH OR BOUILLON CANNED SOUP, READY-TO-SERVE	17	3	1	0	1 CUP

FOODS WITH 0 CARBS

Food Group	Sub-Group	Food Description	Calories	Protein	Fat	Net Carbs	Serving Size
OTHER	SPICES AND HERBS	CAPERS, CANNED	2	0	0	0	1 TBSP.
OTHER	SPICES AND HERBS	CIDER VINEGAR	3	0	0	0	1 TBSP.
OTHER	SPICES AND HERBS	DISTILLED VINEGAR	3	0	0	0	1 TBSP.
OTHER	SPICES AND HERBS	RED WINE VINEGAR	3	0	0	0	1 TBSP.
OTHER	SPICES AND HERBS	SALT, TABLE	0	0	0	0	1 TBSP.
OTHER	SWEETS	GELATINS, DRY POWDER, UNSWEETENED	94	24	0	0	1-1 OZ PACKAGE
OTHER	SWEETS	SWEETENERS, SUGAR SUBSTITUTE, GRANULATED, BROWN	0	0	0	0	1 TSP
PROTEIN	BEEF	BEEF, BRISKET, WHOLE, ALL GRADES, BRAISED	281	22	21	0	3 OZ
PROTEIN	BEEF	BEEF, CURED, CORNED BEEF, BRISKET, COOKED	213	15	16	0	3 OZ
PROTEIN	BEEF	BEEF, GROUND, 70% LEAN MEAT / 30% FAT	211	20	14	0	3 OZ
PROTEIN	BEEF	BEEF, GROUND, 80% LEAN MEAT / 20% FAT	216	21	14	0	3 OZ
PROTEIN	BEEF	BEEF, GROUND, PATTIES, FROZEN, BROILED	251	20	19	0	3 OZ
PROTEIN	BEEF	BEEF, LOIN, TOP LOIN STEAK	224	22	15	0	3 OZ
PROTEIN	BEEF	BEEF, RIB EYE ROAST	248	21	18	0	3 OZ
PROTEIN	BEEF	BEEF, RIB EYE STEAK	247	20	19	0	3 OZ
PROTEIN	BEEF	BEEF, RIB, SHORT RIBS	400	18	36	0	3 OZ
PROTEIN	BEEF	BEEF, RIBS	298	19	24	0	3 OZ
PROTEIN	BEEF	BEEF, ROUND, BOTTOM ROUND, STEAK	210	28	10	0	3 OZ
PROTEIN	BEEF	BEEF, ROUND, EYE OF ROUND, ROAST	177	24	8	0	3 OZ
PROTEIN	BEEF	BEEF, ROUND, TIP ROUND, ROAST	186	23	10	0	3 OZ
PROTEIN	BEEF	BEEF, ROUND, TOP ROUND STEAK	173	26	8	0	3 OZ

FOODS WITH 0 CARBS

Food Group	Sub-Group	Food Description	Calories	Protein	Fat	Net Carbs	Serving Size
PROTEIN	BEEF	BEEF, SHORT LOIN, PORTERHOUSE STEAK	235	22	16	0	3 OZ
PROTEIN	BEEF	BEEF, SHORT LOIN, T-BONE STEAK	246	21	17	0	3 OZ
PROTEIN	BEEF	BEEF, TENDERLOIN, ROAST	275	20	21	0	3 OZ
PROTEIN	BEEF	BEEF, TENDERLOIN, STEAK	227	22	15	0	3 OZ
PROTEIN	BEEF	BEEF, TOP SIRLOIN, STEAK	207	23	12	0	3 OZ
PROTEIN	CHICKEN	CHICKEN, BROILER, ROTISSERIE, BBQ, BACK MEAT AND SKIN	213	17	16	0	3 OZ
PROTEIN	CHICKEN	CHICKEN, BROILER, ROTISSERIE, BBQ, BACK MEAT ONLY	180	19	12	0	3 OZ
PROTEIN	CHICKEN	CHICKEN, BROILER, ROTISSERIE, BBQ, BREAST MEAT AND SKIN	149	22	7	0	3 OZ
PROTEIN	CHICKEN	CHICKEN, BROILER, ROTISSERIE, BBQ, BREAST MEAT ONLY	122	24	3	0	3 OZ
PROTEIN	CHICKEN	CHICKEN, BROILER, ROTISSERIE, BBQ, DRUMSTICK MEAT AND SKIN	146	18	8	0	1 DRUMSTICK
PROTEIN	CHICKEN	CHICKEN, BROILER, ROTISSERIE, BBQ, DRUMSTICK, MEAT ONLY	122	20	5	0	1 DRUMSTICK
PROTEIN	CHICKEN	CHICKEN, BROILER, ROTISSERIE, BBQ, THIGH MEAT AND SKIN	215	21	14	0	1 THIGH
PROTEIN	CHICKEN	CHICKEN, BROILER, ROTISSERIE, BBQ, THIGH, MEAT ONLY	183	23	10	0	1 THIGH
PROTEIN	CHICKEN	CHICKEN, BROILER, ROTISSERIE, BBQ, WING MEAT AND SKIN	131	12	9	0	1 WING
PROTEIN	CHICKEN	CHICKEN, BROILER, ROTISSERIE, BBQ, WING, MEAT ONLY	94	14	4	0	1 WING
PROTEIN	CHICKEN	CHICKEN, BROILERS OR FRYERS, BREAST, MEAT AND SKIN, ROASTED	276	42	11	0	1 CUP

FOODS WITH 0 CARBS

Food Group	Sub-Group	Food Description	Calories	Protein	Fat	Net Carbs	Serving Size
PROTEIN	CHICKEN	CHICKEN, BROILERS OR FRYERS, BREAST, MEAT ONLY, ROASTED	231	43	5	0	1 CUP
PROTEIN	CHICKEN	CHICKEN, BROILERS OR FRYERS, DARK MEAT, DRUMSTICK, MEAT AND SKIN, BRAISED	196	24	11	0	1 DRUMSTICK, WITH SKIN
PROTEIN	CHICKEN	CHICKEN, BROILERS OR FRYERS, DARK MEAT, MEAT AND SKIN, ROASTED	423	43	26	0	1/2 CHICKEN, BONE REMOVED
PROTEIN	CHICKEN	CHICKEN, BROILERS OR FRYERS, DARK MEAT, THIGH, MEAT AND SKIN, BRAISED	295	29	20	0	1 THIGH, WITH SKIN
PROTEIN	CHICKEN	CHICKEN, BROILERS OR FRYERS, DRUMSTICK, MEAT AND SKIN, ROASTED	201	25	11	0	1 DRUMSTICK, WITH SKIN (YIELD FROM 1 LB. READY-TO-COOK CHICKEN)
PROTEIN	CHICKEN	CHICKEN, BROILERS OR FRYERS, LEG, MEAT AND SKIN, ROASTED	156	20	8	0	3 OZ
PROTEIN	CHICKEN	CHICKEN, BROILERS OR FRYERS, LEG, MEAT ONLY, ROASTED	148	21	7	0	3 OZ
PROTEIN	CHICKEN	CHICKEN, BROILERS OR FRYERS, LIGHT MEAT, MEAT AND SKIN, ROASTED	293	38	14	0	1/2 CHICKEN, BONE REMOVED
PROTEIN	CHICKEN	CHICKEN, BROILERS OR FRYERS, LIGHT MEAT, MEAT ONLY, ROASTED	242	43	6	0	1 CUP
PROTEIN	CHICKEN	CHICKEN, BROILERS OR FRYERS, MEAT AND SKIN AND GIBLETS AND NECK, ROASTED	199	23	11	0	3 OZ
PROTEIN	CHICKEN	CHICKEN, BROILERS OR FRYERS, THIGH, MEAT AND SKIN, ROASTED	318	32	20	0	1 THIGH, WITH SKIN
PROTEIN	CHICKEN	CHICKEN, CANNED, MEAT ONLY, WITH BROTH	234	31	11	0	1 CAN, (5 OZ)
PROTEIN	CHICKEN	CHICKEN, DARK MEAT, DRUMSTICK, MEAT AND SKIN, ENHANCED, ROASTED	232	32	12	0	1 DRUMSTICK, WITH SKIN

FOODS WITH 0 CARBS

Food Group	Sub-Group	Food Description	Calories	Protein	Fat	Net Carbs	Serving Size
PROTEIN	CHICKEN	CHICKEN, DARK MEAT, THIGH, MEAT AND SKIN, ENHANCED, ROASTED	278	31	18	0	1 THIGH, WITH SKIN
PROTEIN	CHICKEN	CHICKEN, ROASTING, LIGHT MEAT, MEAT ONLY, ROASTED	214	38	6	0	1 CUP
PROTEIN	CHICKEN	CHICKEN, ROASTING, MEAT AND SKIN AND GIBLETS AND NECK, ROASTED	187	20	11	0	3 OZ
PROTEIN	CHICKEN	CHICKEN, ROASTING, MEAT AND SKIN, ROASTED	190	20	11	0	3 OZ
PROTEIN	CHICKEN	CORNISH GAME HENS, MEAT AND SKIN, ROASTED	220	19	15	0	3 OZ
PROTEIN	EGG	EGG, WHOLE, COOKED, FRIED	90	6	7	0	1 LARGE
PROTEIN	EGG	EGG, WHOLE, COOKED, OMELET	23	2	2	0	1 TBSP.
PROTEIN	EGG	EGG, WHOLE, COOKED, POACHED	72	6	5	0	1 LARGE
PROTEIN	EGG	EGG, WHOLE, COOKED, SCRAMBLED	20	1	2	0	1 TBSP.
PROTEIN	FISH	ANCHOVY, EUROPEAN, CANNED IN OIL, DRAINED SOLIDS	8	1	0	0	1 ANCHOVY
PROTEIN	FISH	BASS, FRESHWATER, MIXED SPECIES	124	21	4	0	3 OZ
PROTEIN	FISH	BASS, STRIPED	105	19	3	0	3 OZ
PROTEIN	FISH	HADDOCK	77	17	0	0	3 OZ
PROTEIN	FISH	HALIBUT, ATLANTIC AND PACIFIC	94	19	1	0	3 OZ
PROTEIN	FISH	HALIBUT, GREENLAND	203	16	15	0	3 OZ
PROTEIN	FISH	ROUGHY, ORANGE	89	19	1	0	3 OZ
PROTEIN	FISH	SALMON, ATLANTIC, FARMED	175	19	10	0	3 OZ
PROTEIN	FISH	SALMON, ATLANTIC, WILD	155	22	7	0	3 OZ
PROTEIN	FISH	SALMON, CHINOOK	196	22	11	0	3 OZ
PROTEIN	FISH	SALMON, CHINOOK, SMOKED	99	16	4	0	3 OZ

FOODS WITH 0 CARBS

Food Group	Sub-Group	Food Description	Calories	Protein	Fat	Net Carbs	Serving Size
PROTEIN	FISH	SALMON, CHINOOK, SMOKED (LOX), REGULAR	33	5	1	0	1 OZ
PROTEIN	FISH	SALMON, PINK	130	21	4	0	3 OZ
PROTEIN	FISH	SALMON, PINK, CANNED, TOTAL CAN CONTENTS	110	17	4	0	3 OZ
PROTEIN	FISH	SALMON, SOCKEYE	144	22	6	0	3 OZ
PROTEIN	FISH	SALMON, SOCKEYE, CANNED, TOTAL CAN CONTENTS	130	18	6	0	3 OZ
PROTEIN	FISH	SARDINE, ATLANTIC, CANNED IN OIL, DRAINED SOLIDS WITH BONE	59	7	3	0	1 OZ
PROTEIN	FISH	SARDINE, PACIFIC, CANNED IN TOMATO SAUCE, DRAINED SOLIDS WITH BONE	165	19	9	0	1 CUP
PROTEIN	FISH	SEA BASS, MIXED SPECIES	105	20	2	0	3 OZ
PROTEIN	FISH	SNAPPER, MIXED SPECIES	109	22	1	0	3 OZ
PROTEIN	FISH	SWORD	146	20	7	0	3 OZ
PROTEIN	FISH	TROUT, MIXED SPECIES	162	23	7	0	3 OZ
PROTEIN	FISH	TROUT, RAINBOW, FARMED	143	20	6	0	3 OZ
PROTEIN	FISH	TROUT, RAINBOW, WILD	128	19	5	0	3 OZ
PROTEIN	FISH	TUNA, FRESH, BLUEFIN	156	25	5	0	3 OZ
PROTEIN	FISH	TUNA, LIGHT, CANNED IN OIL SOLIDS	168	25	7	0	3 OZ
PROTEIN	FISH	TUNA, WHITE, CANNED IN OIL SOLIDS	158	23	7	0	3 OZ
PROTEIN	FISH	TUNA, YELLOWFIN, FRESH	111	25	1	0	3 OZ
PROTEIN	FISH	YELLOWTAIL, MIXED SPECIES	159	25	6	0	3 OZ
PROTEIN	GAME	BISON, GROUND, GRASS-FED, COOKED	152	22	7	0	3 OZ
PROTEIN	GAME	BISON, GROUND, PAN-BROILED	202	20	13	0	3 OZ
PROTEIN	LAMB	LAMB, FORE SHANK, BRAISED	207	24	11	0	3 OZ

FOODS WITH 0 CARBS

Food Group	Sub-Group	Food Description	Calories	Protein	Fat	Net Carbs	Serving Size
PROTEIN	LAMB	LAMB, GROUND, BROILED	241	21	17	0	3 OZ
PROTEIN	LEGUME	SOY PROTEIN ISOLATE	95	23	1	0	1 OZ
PROTEIN	LEGUME	SOY PROTEIN ISOLATE, POTASSIUM TYPE, CRUDE PROTEIN BASIS	90	25	0	0	1 OZ
PROTEIN	LUNCH MEAT	BACON AND BEEF STICKS	145	8	12	0	1 OZ
PROTEIN	LUNCH MEAT	CHICKEN BREAST, DELI, ROTISSERIE SEASONED, SLICED, PREPACKAGED	12	2	0	0	1 SLICE
PROTEIN	LUNCH MEAT	CORNED BEEF LOAF, JELLIED	43	6	2	0	1 SLICE, 4" × 4" × 3/32" THICK
PROTEIN	LUNCH MEAT	HAM, CHOPPED, CANNED	67	4	5	0	1 OZ
PROTEIN	LUNCH MEAT	LEBANON BOLOGNA, BEEF	49	5	3	0	1 OZ
PROTEIN	LUNCH MEAT	PASTRAMI	41	6	2	0	1 SLICE, 1 OZ
PROTEIN	LUNCH MEAT	PEPPERONI, PORK, BEEF	138	6	12	0	1 OZ
PROTEIN	LUNCH MEAT	ROAST BEEF, DELI STYLE, PREPACKAGED, SLICED	10	2	0	0	1 SLICE, OVAL
PROTEIN	LUNCH MEAT	SALAMI, BEEF AND PORK	40	3	3	0	1 SLICE, ROUND
PROTEIN	LUNCH MEAT	SALAMI, DRY OR HARD, PORK, BEEF	106	6	9	0	1 OZ
PROTEIN	LUNCH MEAT	SALAMI, ITALIAN, PORK	119	6	10	0	1 OZ
PROTEIN	LUNCH MEAT	TURKEY BACON, MICROWAVED	29	2	2	0	1 SLICE
PROTEIN	MEAT SUBSTI-TUTE	CHICKEN, MEATLESS	376	40	21	0	1 CUP
PROTEIN	PORK	BACON, PAN-FRIED, BROILED OR ROASTED	172	12	12	0	4 SLICES
PROTEIN	PORK	CANADIAN BACON, PAN-FRIED	19	4	0	0	1 SLICE
PROTEIN	PORK	HAM WITH NATURAL JUICES, PAN-BROIL	153	22	7	0	3 OZ
PROTEIN	PORK	PORK FEET, PICKLED	39	3	3	0	1 OZ
PROTEIN	PORK	PORK, BACK RIBS, ROASTED	248	20	18	0	3 OZ

FOODS WITH 0 CARBS

Food Group	Sub-Group	Food Description	Calories	Protein	Fat	Net Carbs	Serving Size
PROTEIN	PORK	PORK, LOIN, BLADE (CHOPS)	196	20	12	0	3 OZ
PROTEIN	PORK	PORK, LOIN, BLADE (ROASTS)	169	23	9	0	3 OZ
PROTEIN	PORK	PORK, LOIN, CENTER LOIN (CHOPS)	178	22	9	0	3 OZ
PROTEIN	PORK	PORK, LOIN, CENTER LOIN (ROASTS)	196	23	11	0	3 OZ
PROTEIN	PORK	PORK, LOIN, CENTER RIB (CHOPS)	221	23	13	0	3 OZ
PROTEIN	PORK	PORK, LOIN, CENTER RIB (ROASTS)	214	23	13	0	3 OZ
PROTEIN	PORK	PORK, LOIN, COUNTRY-STYLE RIBS	301	32	19	0	1 RACK
PROTEIN	PORK	PORK, LOIN, TENDERLOIN	171	25	7	0	3 OZ
PROTEIN	PORK	PORK, LOIN, TOP LOIN (CHOPS)	167	23	8	0	3 OZ
PROTEIN	PORK	PORK, LOIN, TOP LOIN (ROASTS)	163	22	7	0	3 OZ
PROTEIN	PORK	PORK, LOIN, WHOLE	206	23	12	0	3 OZ
PROTEIN	PORK	PORK, SHOULDER BREAST	138	24	4	0	3 OZ
PROTEIN	PORK	PORK, SHOULDER, WHOLE, ROASTED	248	20	18	0	3 OZ
PROTEIN	PORK	PORK, SPARERIBS	307	18	26	0	3 OZ
PROTEIN	SAUSAGE	BEEF SAUSAGE, FRESH, COOKED	143	8	12	0	1 SERVING
PROTEIN	SAUSAGE	BEEF SAUSAGE, PRE-COOKED	194	7	18	0	1 SERVING
PROTEIN	SAUSAGE	PORK SAUSAGE, LINK/PATTY, FULLY MICROWAVED	92	3	9	0	1 LINK
PROTEIN	SAUSAGE	PORK SAUSAGE, LINK/PATTY, PAN-FRIED	75	4	6	0	1 LINK
PROTEIN	SAUSAGE	SAUSAGE, CHICKEN AND BEEF, SMOKED	407	26	33	0	1 CUP
PROTEIN	SAUSAGE	TURKEY SAUSAGE, FRESH, COOKED	112	14	6	0	1 SERVING
PROTEIN	SEED	FLAXSEED	53	2	4	0	1 TBSP.

FOODS WITH 0 CARBS

Food Group	Sub-Group	Food Description	Calories	Protein	Fat	Net Carbs	Serving Size
PROTEIN	SHELLFISH	CRAB, ALASKA KING	82	16	1	0	3 OZ
PROTEIN	SHELLFISH	LOBSTER, NORTHERN	76	16	1	0	3 OZ
PROTEIN	TURKEY	GROUND TURKEY, 85% LEAN, 15% FAT	219	21	15	0	3 OZ
PROTEIN	TURKEY	TURKEY BREAST, PRE-BASTED, MEAT AND SKIN, ROASTED	107	19	3	0	3 OZ
PROTEIN	TURKEY	TURKEY THIGH, PRE-BASTED, MEAT AND SKIN, ROASTED	133	16	7	0	3 OZ
PROTEIN	TURKEY	TURKEY, ALL CLASSES, BACK, MEAT AND SKIN, ROASTED	342	37	20	0	1 CUP
PROTEIN	TURKEY	TURKEY, BREAST, FROM WHOLE BIRD, ENHANCED, MEAT ONLY, ROASTED	108	23	2	0	3 OZ
PROTEIN	TURKEY	TURKEY, BREAST, FROM WHOLE BIRD, NON-ENHANCED, MEAT ONLY, ROASTED	125	26	2	0	3 OZ
PROTEIN	TURKEY	TURKEY, BREAST, MEAT AND SKIN, ROASTED	139	25	5	0	3 OZ
PROTEIN	TURKEY	TURKEY, DRUMSTICK, FROM WHOLE BIRD, MEAT ONLY, ROASTED	118	26	2	0	3 OZ
PROTEIN	TURKEY	TURKEY, FRYER-ROASTERS, MEAT AND SKIN, ROASTED	146	24	5	0	3 OZ
PROTEIN	TURKEY	TURKEY, RETAIL PARTS, DRUMSTICK, MEAT AND SKIN, ROASTED	167	24	8	0	3 OZ
PROTEIN	TURKEY	TURKEY, RETAIL PARTS, ENHANCED, BREAST, MEAT ONLY, ROASTED	111	24	2	0	3 OZ
PROTEIN	TURKEY	TURKEY, RETAIL PARTS, THIGH, MEAT AND SKIN, ROASTED	156	20	8	0	3 OZ
PROTEIN	TURKEY	TURKEY, RETAIL PARTS, WING, MEAT AND SKIN, ROASTED	200	24	11	0	3 OZ
PROTEIN	TURKEY	TURKEY, WHOLE, ENHANCED, MEAT AND SKIN, ROASTED	150	22	7	0	3 OZ

FOODS WITH 0 CARBS

Food Group	Sub-Group	Food Description	Calories	Protein	Fat	Net Carbs	Serving Size
PROTEIN	TURKEY	TURKEY, WHOLE, MEAT AND SKIN, ROASTED	161	24	6	0	3 OZ
PROTEIN	VEAL	VEAL, FORE SHANK, OSSO BUCO, BRAISED	155	24	7	0	3 OZ
PROTEIN	VEAL	VEAL, GROUND	146	21	6	0	3 OZ
PROTEIN	VEAL	VEAL, LOIN, CHOP, GRILLED	168	24	8	0	3 OZ
PROTEIN	VEAL	VEAL, LOIN, ROASTED	184	21	10	0	3 OZ
PROTEIN	VEAL	VEAL, SIRLOIN, ROASTED	172	21	9	0	3 OZ
VEGETABLE	VEGETABLE	ALFALFA SEEDS, SPROUTED, RAW	8	1	0	0	1 CUP
VEGETABLE	VEGETABLE	ARUGULA, RAW	3	0	0	0	1/2 CUP
VEGETABLE	VEGETABLE	ASPARAGUS, COOKED	32	5	1	0	1 CUP
VEGETABLE	VEGETABLE	BROCCOLI RAAB, RAW	9	1	0	0	1 CUP
VEGETABLE	VEGETABLE	CHARD, SWISS, RAW	7	1	0	0	1 CUP
VEGETABLE	VEGETABLE	ENDIVE, RAW	4	0	0	0	1/2 CUP
VEGETABLE	VEGETABLE	FUNGI, CLOUD EARS, DRIED	80	3	0	0	1 CUP
VEGETABLE	VEGETABLE	GINGER ROOT, RAW	2	0	0	0	1 TSP
VEGETABLE	VEGETABLE	KALE, RAW	8	1	0	0	1 CUP
VEGETABLE	VEGETABLE	LETTUCE, BUTTERHEAD (INCLUDES BOSTON AND BIBB TYPES), RAW	7	1	0	0	1 CUP
VEGETABLE	VEGETABLE	ONIONS, YOUNG GREEN, TOPS ONLY	2	0	0	0	1 TBSP.
VEGETABLE	VEGETABLE	PEPPERS, HOT CHILE, SUN-DRIED	2	0	0	0	1 PEPPER
VEGETABLE	VEGETABLE	PICKLES, CUCUMBER, DILL OR KOSHER DILL	1	0	0	0	1 SLICE
VEGETABLE	VEGETABLE	SPINACH, RAW	7	1	0	0	1 CUP
VEGETABLE	VEGETABLE	WATERCRESS, RAW	4	1	0	0	1 CUP

How Much Protein Should You Eat?

Take a look at your body composition results and determine your lean body mass—the weight of your muscle and bones. Your protein rations in the five-week metabolic makeover plan are generally determined by your lean body weight or fat-free mass. So if you're 150 pounds and have 30 percent fat, you will have 45 pounds of fat weight and 105 pounds of lean mass. Use that 105 pounds of lean mass to calculate your protein requirement. I advise that you construct your protein levels based on 1 gram of protein per pound of lean body mass or weight. In the above 150-pound person that would translate into approximately 105 grams of protein a day. Some might think this is a high number, but if you are engaging in muscle building activity like we are with our high intensity SMaRT exercise sessions, some extra protein may be necessary. The above carbohydrate charts also include protein grams, so you can use these to calculate your daily protein intake as well.

How Much Fat Should You Eat?

The remainder of your food and caloric intake should come from fats. So let's imagine that you're taking in 40 grams of carbs per day. That's about 160 calories. Next, let's assume that you're taking in 100 grams of protein per day. That's about 400 calories. The rest of your caloric consumption will be derived from fat (probably anywhere from 80 to 150 grams of fat). That's about 640 to 1,200 calories from fat. That's assuming that you are moderately active and trying to lose fat. Remember that the body weight that was used to calculate this general formula is about 150 pounds. The preceding food charts provide fat content in many portions of many foods.

Remember, the carbohydrate levels do not really fluctuate with body size or even lean tissue weight very much. The protein intake can vary greatly, depending upon overall size and especially lean tissue weight. Lastly, the fat content or amount of fat eaten can vary enormously, depending upon activity levels, appetite, and amount of fat to be lost on your plan. Don't try to cut back severely on carbohydrates *and* fat. It will leave you with a very high protein diet, which admittedly works for quite a few folks but may impede lean tissue levels—not by a shortage of available protein but a shortage of energy necessary to fuel muscle-building activity. These "manipulations" in dietary plans and nutritional content are a highly personal, subjective process and should be closely monitored to direct any individual adjustments. However, these guidelines are certainly historically healthy for most people and hopefully you can find a doctor who understands the basic physiology and metabolic consequences involved.

Good Fats

As a word of encouragement and reinforcement for eating more fat than is conventionally recommended, let me remind you: 100 million Americans are overweight, and that number increases significantly every year and has since we were told to cut back on fats. Why is this bad? Because increased weight increases mortality for all causes. Additionally, if you suffer from one or more of these symptoms, it can quite likely be a result of eating too little fat: weight gain, fatigue, consistent hunger, cravings, hormone problems, an uncontrollable "sweet tooth," and the seeming impossibility of getting those last few pounds off regardless of serious calorie reduction.

Here's a simple description of fats:

- **Saturated fats:** These are mainly animal fats, usually solid at room temperature. They are great at providing satiety (fullness). These have been demonized as "bad," causing health problems, including high cholesterol. None of these criticisms are scientifically valid. Saturated fats include butter, red meats and poultry, cheese, heavy cream, nuts, and even some processed meats like pepperoni.

- **Omega-3 fatty acids:** These include egg yolks, cod liver oil and flax oil, meats, and dairy products.

- **Medium-chain fatty acids (MCFAs):** MCFAs are interesting fats. They are hard to store and are quick to be used as energy—great for reducing stored body fat and satisfying hunger. Coconut oil is an MCFA, and the more you take in, the fewer essential omegas you need to do the job.

- **Monosaturated or Monounsaturated fats:** These are the famous good "Mediterranean" fats and include olive oil, canola oil, peanut oil, safflower oil, sesame oil, avocados, peanut butter (careful of "added" sugar), many other nuts, butter, eggs, cheeses, and fish (salmon, halibut, mackerel, sable and herring).

Fruits and Vegetables

These two categories of food are almost always mentioned in the same breath. The government does it. Doctors do it. Health and diet books do it. It's CRAZY! Fruit, even from the Garden of Eden, is Mother Nature's candy. It is full of a sugar called fructose. An irrational attachment to the idea of the "wonderfulness" of fruit still exists. In the developmental history of the human genetics, fruits were not often available (seasonal at best) and were certainly not as "sugary" as our modern day, cultivated versions of the originals.

Many of us are "carbohydrate sensitive." That means that sugar, in any form, causes us to respond in a way that overproduces insulin, the hormone that drives fat storage and accumulation. Be it a Snickers bar, an orange, a piece of birthday cake, or a peach, sugar is sugar and follows a similar pathway in our metabolism despite its source.

The difference between fruits and vegetables is simply night and day, nutritionally. Vegetables are much lower in calorie and carbohydrate density than fruits. Think of the difference between a garden salad full of different types of lettuces and greens and a fruit salad containing a variety of fruits. The difference in calorie content can easily be ten times for the fruit than veggie version. Causing that discrepancy is the sugar content. The takeaway is that vegetables are good, and fruits, not so much for those watching their sugar intake.

The SMaRT Eating Plan Works!

Mo was a 50-year-old woman who was athletic and always in shape. She was constantly active and fairly disciplined with her eating. As a result, she never had a weight problem *until* she reached the magic 50. Things began to change, and for the first time weight just accumulated, much to her dismay. She went to a few doctors and they tried to fiddle with her hormones, checking her thyroid, among other possibilities, all to no avail.

About 18 months into this problematic state, Mo was having some respiratory issues, and her doctor (separately and distinctively of her weight problem) advised her that she should cut way back on sugar (carbs), since he diagnosed her with an anaerobic allergy condition. So Mo cut down severely on all carbohydrates and—like magic!—her weight began to drop. When I saw her after about six weeks on the "no sugar" diet (or something very close), she really looked 10 years younger and had regained her athletic physique and childish behavior (that's an inside joke between Mo and me).

5 Steps to SMaRT Success

1. **Get organized.** Most people haven't really analyzed their eating patterns. How many carbohydrates are you eating? What are the glycemic indexes and loads ("sugar effects") of those? How much protein are you eating and how much fat? Learn how to read labels and figure out exactly what you're eating.

2. **Be prepared.** Make a list of the foods you want to eat that fit into your guidelines and stock your fridge and pantry with them. Don't be hesitant to eat any acceptable food at any time of the day. For example, if you want to eat chicken for breakfast, go ahead. If you want eggs for dinner, so be it. Just have the right foods around to eat so that you don't have to compromise your plan.

3. **Record your efforts.** I've been doing this personally for more than 30 years. You'd be surprised how simply writing down everything you eat and drink each day makes you tow the line, being accountable to yourself. This practice helps analyze pitfalls and habits that may jeopardize your progress.

4. **Get up when you fall.** This weight-loss process almost never goes without a bump or hurdle. In fact, statistics indicate that people who finally succeed at keeping weight off have tried multiple times before they finally achieve that goal. Don't allow one misstep to derail your progress; get right back on your plan.

5. **Believe.** The information you've been reading in this book provides you with the best, most practical, and long-term effective chance of getting where you belong and want to be. There's nothing sold here, no miracles or potions, only a solid, safe plan that has proven to be effective for many thousands of folks just like you and me!

It's not magic, but sometimes just the simple yet significant reduction in refined sugars and simple carbohydrates (low carb) can make all the difference in the world for both health and cosmetic problems. Combined with the SMaRT exercise plan, this is the most consistently successful, long-term answer for fat-related conditions and turns that status around very quickly.

Five Weeks of Daily SMaRT Meal Plans

CAVEAT: *The following meal plans are simply suggestions for average-sized people with an average body composition. Some meals might be right up your alley, and you'll want to eat them regularly, and some you might exclude from your menu immediately. The carbohydrate total is the important number. That has very little "wiggle room." The fat count can be readily increased and the protein content can be manipulated 10 percent to 20 percent in most cases.* **REMEMBER**, *if you like certain meals you can eat them for breakfast, lunch, or dinner day after day. Just be cognizant of the general guidelines and selections.*

DAILY SMART MEAL PLANS

Day	Meal	Food Description	Calories	Proteins	Fat	Net Carbs	Serving Size
		WEEK ONE					
1	BREAKFAST	CHEESE, MONTEREY	421	28	34	1	1 CUP, CUBED
1	BREAKFAST	TEA, BLACK, BREWED	2	0	0	1	6 FL OZ
1	BREAKFAST	CREAM, HEAVY	104	0	12	0	2 TBSP.
1	BREAKFAST	TOTAL	527	28	46	2	
1	LUNCH	**HAM WRAP**					
1	LUNCH	▷ HAM, SLICED, REGULAR	184	20	8	4	4 SLICES
1	LUNCH	▷ CHEESE, CHEDDAR	220	14	18	4	2 OZ
1	LUNCH	▷ TORTILLAS, LOW CARB, WHOLE WHEAT, FLOUR	90	3	2	3	1 TORTILLA, 28G
1	LUNCH	TEA, BLACK, BREWED	2	0	0	1	6 FL OZ
1	LUNCH	CREAM, HEAVY	104	0	12	0	2 TBSP.
1	LUNCH	TOTAL	600	37	40	12	
1	DINNER	**BEEF, RIB EYE STEAK**	247	20	19	0	3 OZ
1	DINNER	**SPINACH SALAD**					
1	DINNER	▷ SPINACH, RAW	7	1	0	0	1 CUP
1	DINNER	▷ SALAD DRESSING, BACON AND TOMATO	49	0	5	0	1 TBSP.
1	DINNER	▷ CHEESE, GOAT, HARD TYPE	127	9	10	1	1 OZ
1	DINNER	▷ ALMONDS, DRY ROASTED	413	15	37	7	1/2 CUP
1	DINNER	▷ AVOCADOS, RAW, CALIFORNIA	192	3	17.5	2	1/2 CUP
1	DINNER	▷ MUSHROOMS, WHITE, RAW	21	3	0	2	1 CUP
1	DINNER	▷ STRAWBERRIES, RAW	37	1	1	7	1/2 CUP
1	DINNER	WINE, TABLE, WHITE, CHARDONNAY	123	0	0	3	5 FL OZ

DAILY SMART MEAL PLANS

Day	Meal	Food Description	Calories	Proteins	Fat	Net Carbs	Serving Size
1	DINNER	TOTAL	1216	52	89.5	22	
2	BREAKFAST	**MEATLESS BACON WRAP**					
2	BREAKFAST	▷ BACON, MEATLESS	446	15	43	5	1 CUP
2	BREAKFAST	▷ TORTILLAS, LOW CARB, WHOLE WHEAT, FLOUR	90	3	2	3	1 TORTILLA, 28G
2	BREAKFAST	▷ CHEESE, MONTEREY	211	14	17	1	4 OZ
2	BREAKFAST	HIBISCUS TEA	0	0	0	0	8 FL OZ
2	BREAKFAST	TOTAL	747	32	62	9	
2	LUNCH	**CHICKEN, MEATLESS**	376	40	21	0	1 CUP
2	LUNCH	CRACKERS, LOW CARB	100	4	7	6	10 CRACKERS
2	LUNCH	CHEESE, PARMESAN, GRATED	42	2	2	2	2 TBSP.
2	LUNCH	TEA, BLACK, BREWED, ICED	2	0	0	1	8 FL OZ
2	LUNCH	TOTAL	520	46	30	9	
2	DINNER	**VEGGIE BURGER**					
2	DINNER	▷ VEGGIE BURGERS OR SOY BURGERS, UNPREPARED	124	11	4	7	1 PATTY
2	DINNER	▷ OIL, COCONUT	112	0	13	0	1 TBSP.
2	DINNER	▷ BARBECUE SAUCE	29	0	0	7	1 TBSP.
2	DINNER	▷ MAYONNAISE DRESSING	103	0	12	0	1 TBSP.
2	DINNER	▷ BREAD, LOW CARB	120	12	4	2	2 SLICE, 1 OZ
2	DINNER	▷ CHEESE, CHEDDAR	440	28	36	8	4 OZ
2	DINNER	WATER	0	0	0	0	8 FL OZ
2	DINNER	TOTAL	928	51	69	24	
3	BREAKFAST	WALNUTS, ENGLISH	381	9	38	8	1/2 CUP
3	BREAKFAST	CHEESE, COTTAGE, CREAMED, LARGE OR SMALL CURD	111	13	5	4	4 OZ

DAILY SMART MEAL PLANS

Day	Meal	Food Description	Calories	Proteins	Fat	Net Carbs	Serving Size
3	BREAKFAST	COFFEE, BREWED FROM GROUNDS, PREPARED WITH TAP WATER	0	0	0	0	6 FL OZ
3	BREAKFAST	TOTAL	492	22	43	12	
3	LUNCH	**TEMPEH STIR-FRY**					
3	LUNCH	▷ TEMPEH	346	34	12	6	6 OZ
3	LUNCH	▷ ASPARAGUS, COOKED	32	5	1	0	1 CUP
3	LUNCH	▷ OIL, OLIVE, SALAD OR COOKING	230	0	26	0	2 TBSP.
3	LUNCH	▷ SOY SAUCE MADE FROM SOY (TAMARI)	22	4	0	2	1 TBSP.
3	LUNCH	COFFEE, BREWED FROM GROUNDS, PREPARED WITH TAP WATER	0	0	0	0	6 FL OZ
3	LUNCH	CREAM, HEAVY	104	0	12	0	2 TBSP.
3	LUNCH	TOTAL	734	43	51	8	
3	DINNER	HAM, SLICE, BONE-IN, PAN-BROIL	306	44	14	2	6 OZ
3	DINNER	ASPARAGUS, COOKED	32	5	1	0	1 CUP
3	DINNER	BUTTER, SALTED	102	0	12	0	1 TBSP.
3	DINNER	CHEESE, PARMESAN, GRATED	84	4	4	4	4 TBSP.
3	DINNER	CARBONATED BEVERAGE, 0 CALORIE, ANY FLAVOR	0	0	0	0	12 FL OZ
3	DINNER	DISTILLED, RUM, 80 PROOF	97	0	0	0	1 JIGGER, 1/2 FL OZ
3	DINNER	TOTAL	621	53	31	6	
4	BREAKFAST	CHEESE, SWISS	502	36	37	7	1 CUP, CUBED
4	BREAKFAST	PECANS, DRY ROASTED	199	3	21	1	1 OZ
4	BREAKFAST	WATER	0	0	0	0	8 FL OZ
4	BREAKFAST	TOTAL	701	39	58	8	

DAILY SMART MEAL PLANS

Day	Meal	Food Description	Calories	Proteins	Fat	Net Carbs	Serving Size
4	LUNCH	**BURGER WRAP**					
4	LUNCH	▷ BEEF, GROUND, 70% LEAN MEAT / 30% FAT	211	20	14	0	3 OZ
4	LUNCH	▷ CHEESE, CHEDDAR	220	14	18	4	2 OZ
4	LUNCH	▷ BACON, PAN-FRIED, MICROWAVED OR ROASTED	43	3	3	0	1 SLICE
4	LUNCH	▷ ONIONS, COOKED	14	0	0	4	2 TBSP.
4	LUNCH	▷ MAYONNAISE DRESSING	206	0	24	0	2 TBSP.
4	LUNCH	▷ LETTUCE, BUTTERHEAD (INCLUDES BOSTON AND BIBB TYPES), RAW	7	1	0	0	1 CUP
4	LUNCH	WATER	0	0	0	0	8 FL OZ
4	*LUNCH*	*TOTAL*	*701*	*38*	*59*	*8*	
4	DINNER	**BRATS AND KRAUT**					
4	DINNER	▷ BRATWURST, BEEF AND PORK, SMOKED	196	8	17	1	2-1/3 OZ
4	DINNER	▷ MUSTARD, YELLOW, PREPARED	6	0	0	0	2 TSP
4	DINNER	▷ BREAD, LOW CARB	120	12	4	2	2 SLICE, 1 OZ
4	DINNER	▷ SAUERKRAUT, CANNED, SOLIDS AND LIQUIDS	45	2	0	3	1 CUP
4	DINNER	**SALAD**					
4	DINNER	▷ LETTUCE, BUTTERHEAD (INCLUDES BOSTON AND BIBB TYPES), RAW	7	1	0	0	1 CUP
4	DINNER	▷ SALAD DRESSING, ITALIAN DRESSING	41	0	4	1	1 TBSP.
4	DINNER	▷ WALNUTS, BLACK, DRIED	387	15	37	2	1/2 CUP
4	DINNER	▷ TOMATOES, RED, RAW	32	2	0	5	1 CUP
4	DINNER	WATER	0	0	0	0	8 FL OZ
4	*DINNER*	*TOTAL*	*834*	*40*	*62*	*14*	

DAILY SMART MEAL PLANS

Day	Meal	Food Description	Calories	Proteins	Fat	Net Carbs	Serving Size
5	BREAKFAST	**CHICKEN LETTUCE WRAP**					
5	BREAKFAST	▷ SAUSAGE, CHICKEN AND BEEF, SMOKED	407	26	33	0	1 CUP
5	BREAKFAST	▷ LETTUCE, BUTTERHEAD (INCLUDES BOSTON AND BIBB TYPES), RAW	7	1	0	0	1 CUP
5	BREAKFAST	WATER	0	0	0	0	8 FL OZ
5	*BREAKFAST*	*TOTAL*	*414*	*27*	*33*	*0*	
5	LUNCH	**TUNA SANDWICH**					
5	LUNCH	▷ TUNA, WHITE, CANNED IN OIL SOLIDS	158	23	7	0	3 OZ
5	LUNCH	▷ MAYONNAISE DRESSING	103	0	12	0	1 TBSP.
5	LUNCH	▷ BREAD, LOW CARB	120	12	4	2	2 SLICE, 1 OZ
5	LUNCH	▷ PICKLE RELISH, SWEET	20	0	0	5	1 TBSP.
5	LUNCH	HIBISCUS TEA	0	0	0	0	8 FL OZ
5	*LUNCH*	*TOTAL*	*401*	*35*	*23*	*7*	
5	DINNER	SALMON, ATLANTIC, WILD	310	44	14	0	6 OZ
5	DINNER	BUTTER, WHIPPED	67	0	8	0	1 TBSP.
5	DINNER	**BROCCOLI WITH CHEESE SAUCE**					
5	DINNER	▷ BROCCOLI, COOKED	54	4	0	6	1 CUP
5	DINNER	▷ CHEESE SAUCE, READY-TO-SERVE	110	4	8	4	1/4 CUP
5	DINNER	▷ WHOLE MILK, 3.25% MILKFAT	149	8	8	12	1 CUP
5	*DINNER*	*TOTAL*	*690*	*60*	*38*	*22*	
6	BREAKFAST	**PEANUT BUTTER WRAP**					
6	BREAKFAST	▷ PEANUT BUTTER, CHUNK STYLE	376	16	32	8	4 TBSP.
6	BREAKFAST	▷ TORTILLAS, LOW CARB, WHOLE WHEAT, FLOUR	90	3	2	3	1 TORTILLA, 28G

DAILY SMART MEAL PLANS

Day	Meal	Food Description	Calories	Proteins	Fat	Net Carbs	Serving Size
6	BREAKFAST	▷ CHEESE, MOZZARELLA, WHOLE MILK	85	6	6	1	1 OZ
6	BREAKFAST	▷ TEA, BLACK, BREWED, ICED	2	0	0	1	8 FL OZ
6	*BREAKFAST*	*TOTAL*	*553*	*25*	*40*	*13*	
6	LUNCH	CHICKEN, BROILER, ROTISSERIE, GRILLED, DRUMSTICK MEAT AND SKIN	146	18	8	0	1 DRUMSTICK
6	LUNCH	**SALAD**					
6	LUNCH	▷ LETTUCE, BUTTERHEAD (INCLUDES BOSTON AND BIBB TYPES), RAW	7	1	0	0	1 CUP
6	LUNCH	▷ TOMATOES, RED CHERRY, RAW	27	1	0	4	1 CUP
6	LUNCH	▷ ALMONDS, OIL ROASTED	477	17	44	6	1/2 CUP
6	LUNCH	▷ CHEESE, FETA	75	4	6	1	1 OZ
6	LUNCH	▷ SALAD DRESSING, ITALIAN DRESSING	41	0	4	1	1 TBSP.
6	LUNCH	WATER	0	0	0	0	8 FL OZ
6	*LUNCH*	*TOTAL*	*773*	*41*	*62*	*12*	
6	DINNER	CHICKEN, BROILER, ROTISSERIE, GRILLED, BREAST MEAT AND SKIN	298	44	14	0	6 OZ
6	DINNER	**SALAD**					
6	DINNER	▷ LETTUCE, BUTTERHEAD (INCLUDES BOSTON AND BIBB TYPES), RAW	7	1	0	0	1 CUP
6	DINNER	▷ KALE, RAW	8	1	0	0	1 CUP
6	DINNER	▷ ARUGULA, RAW	3	0	0	0	1/2 CUP
6	DINNER	▷ PECANS, OIL ROASTED	394	5	42	2	1/2 CUP
6	DINNER	▷ CUCUMBER, PEELED, RAW	16	1	0	2	1 CUP
6	DINNER	▷ MUSHROOMS, WHITE, RAW	21	3	0	2	1 CUP
6	DINNER	▷ TOMATOES, RED, RAW	32	2	0	5	1 CUP

DAILY SMART MEAL PLANS

Day	Meal	Food Description	Calories	Proteins	Fat	Net Carbs	Serving Size
6	DINNER	▷ PEPPERS, SWEET, RED, RAW	46	1	0	6	1 CUP
6	DINNER	▷ OIL, AVOCADO	124	0	14	0	1 TBSP.
6	DINNER	▷ BALSAMIC VINEGAR	14	0	0	3	1 TBSP.
6	DINNER	TEA, BLACK, BREWED, ICED	2	0	0	1	8 FL OZ
6	DINNER	TOTAL	965	58	70	21	
7	BREAKFAST	**EGG AND SAUSAGE WRAP**					
7	BREAKFAST	▷ SMOKED LINK SAUSAGE, PORK	420	16	38	2	2 LINK, (4" LONG × 1-1/8" DIA)
7	BREAKFAST	▷ EGG, WHOLE, COOKED, SCRAMBLED	188	12	12	0	4 OZ
7	BREAKFAST	▷ BUTTER, SALTED	102	0	12	0	1 TBSP.
7	BREAKFAST	▷ TORTILLAS, LOW CARB, WHOLE WHEAT, FLOUR	90	3	2	3	1 TORTILLA, 28G
7	BREAKFAST	COCONUT WATER (LIQUID FROM COCONUTS)	46	2	0	6	1 CUP
7	BREAKFAST	TOTAL	846	33	64	11	
7	LUNCH	**SPINACH SALAD**					
7	LUNCH	▷ EGG, WHOLE, COOKED, HARD-BOILED	211	17	14	2	1 CUP
7	LUNCH	▷ SPINACH, RAW	28	4	0	0	4 CUP
7	LUNCH	▷ TOMATOES, YELLOW, RAW	11	1	0	2	1/2 CUP
7	LUNCH	▷ BROCCOLI, FLOWER CLUSTERS, RAW	20	2	0	3	1 CUP
7	LUNCH	▷ PECANS, DRY ROASTED	199	3	21	1	1 OZ
7	LUNCH	▷ CHEESE, MONTEREY	421	28	34	1	1 CUP, CUBED
7	LUNCH	▷ SALAD DRESSING, BLUE OR ROQUEFORT CHEESE DRESSING	292	0	32	4	4 TBSP.
7	LUNCH	WATER	0	0	0	0	8 FL OZ
7	LUNCH	TOTAL	1,182	55	101	13	

DAILY SMART MEAL PLANS

Day	Meal	Food Description	Calories	Proteins	Fat	Net Carbs	Serving Size
7	DINNER	BEEF, SHORT LOIN, T-BONE STEAK	492	42	34	0	6 OZ
7	DINNER	ARTICHOKES (GLOBE OR FRENCH), COOKED	64	3	0	4	1 ARTICHOKE, MEDIUM
7	DINNER	CARROTS, COOKED	54	2	0	8	1 CUP
7	DINNER	BUTTER, SALTED	204	0	24	0	2 TBSP.
7	DINNER	SPARKLING WATER	0	0	0	0	8 FL OZ
7	*DINNER*	*TOTAL*	*814*	*47*	*58*	*12*	

WEEK TWO

Day	Meal	Food Description	Calories	Proteins	Fat	Net Carbs	Serving Size
8	BREAKFAST	**EGG AND SAUSAGE WRAP**					
8	BREAKFAST	▷ SAUSAGE, TURKEY, BREAKFAST LINKS, MILD	264	18	20	2	2 OZ, 4 LINKS
8	BREAKFAST	▷ EGG, WHOLE, COOKED, FRIED	180	12	14	0	2 LARGE
8	BREAKFAST	▷ OIL, OLIVE, SALAD OR COOKING	115	0	13	0	1 TBSP.
8	BREAKFAST	▷ TORTILLAS, LOW CARB, WHOLE WHEAT, FLOUR	90	3	2	3	1 TORTILLA, 28G
8	BREAKFAST	WATER	0	0	0	0	8 FL OZ
8	*BREAKFAST*	*TOTAL*	*649*	*33*	*49*	*5*	
8	LUNCH	SALMON, PINK	260	42	8	0	6 OZ
8	LUNCH	BROCCOLI, CHOPPED, COOKED	52	6	0	4	1 CUP
8	LUNCH	BUTTER, SALTED	204	0	24	0	2 TBSP.
8	LUNCH	TEA, BLACK, BREWED	2	0	0	1	6 FL OZ
8	LUNCH	CREAM, HEAVY	104	0	12	0	2 TBSP.
8	*LUNCH*	*TOTAL*	*622*	*48*	*44*	*5*	

DAILY SMART MEAL PLANS

Day	Meal	Food Description	Calories	Proteins	Fat	Net Carbs	Serving Size
8	DINNER	**HOT DOGS**					
8	DINNER	▷ FRANKFURTER, BEEF AND PORK	274	10	24	2	2 FRANK-FURTER
8	DINNER	▷ PICKLE RELISH, HOT DOG	28	0	0	8	2 TBSP.
8	DINNER	▷ ONIONS, RAW	23	1	0	5	1/2 CUP
8	DINNER	▷ CHEESE, GRUYERE	464	32	36	0	4 OZ
8	DINNER	▷ BREAD, LOW CARB	120	12	4	2	2 SLICE, 1 OZ
8	DINNER	▷ OLIVES, RIPE, CANNED	92	0	8	4	4 OZ
8	DINNER	SPARKLING WATER	0	0	0	0	8 FL OZ
8	DINNER	TOTAL	1,001	55	72	21	
9	BREAKFAST	YOGURT, GREEK, PLAIN, WHOLE MILK	190	18	10	8	1 CUP
9	BREAKFAST	RASPBERRIES, RAW	16	1	1	2	1/4 CUP
9	BREAKFAST	PECANS, OIL ROASTED	404	6	42	2	2 OZ
9	BREAKFAST	TEA, BLACK, BREWED	2	0	0	1	6 FL OZ
9	BREAKFAST	CREAM, HEAVY	104	0	12	0	2 TBSP.
9	BREAKFAST	TOTAL	716	25	65	13	
9	LUNCH	**CHICKEN WRAP**					
9	LUNCH	▷ CHICKEN BREAST, DELI, ROTISSERIE SEASONED, SLICED, PREPACKAGED	96	16	0	0	8 SLICES
9	LUNCH	▷ CHEESE, SWISS	251	18	19	4	1/2 CUP, CUBED
9	LUNCH	▷ LETTUCE, GREEN LEAF, RAW	5	0	0	1	1 CUP
9	LUNCH	▷ MAYONNAISE DRESSING	103	0	12	0	1 TBSP.
9	LUNCH	▷ TORTILLAS, LOW CARB, WHOLE WHEAT, FLOUR	90	3	2	3	1 TORTILLA, 28G

DAILY SMART MEAL PLANS

Day	Meal	Food Description	Calories	Proteins	Fat	Net Carbs	Serving Size
9	LUNCH	TEA, BLACK, BREWED, ICED	2	0	0	1	8 FL OZ
9	LUNCH	TOTAL	547	37	33	9	
9	DINNER	**CANADIAN BACON SANDWICH**					
9	DINNER	▷ CANADIAN BACON, PAN-FRIED	178	24	8	2	4 SLICES
9	DINNER	▷ LETTUCE, GREEN LEAF, RAW	5	0	0	1	1 CUP
9	DINNER	▷ TOMATOES, RED, RAW	32	2	0	5	1 CUP
9	DINNER	▷ MAYONNAISE DRESSING	103	0	12	0	1 TBSP.
9	DINNER	▷ BEANS, SNAP, GREEN, COOKED	38	2	0	5	1 CUP
9	DINNER	▷ BUTTER, SALTED	204	0	24	0	2 TBSP.
9	DINNER	▷ ALMONDS, DRY ROASTED	413	15	37	7	1/2 CUP
9	DINNER	BREAD, LOW CARB	120	12	4	2	2 SLICE, 1 OZ
9	DINNER	TEA, BLACK, BREWED	2	0	0	1	6 FL OZ
9	DINNER	TOTAL	1,095	55	85	23	
9	DINNER	GREEN BEANS AND ALMONDS					
10	BREAKFAST	**TUNA SANDWICH**					
10	BREAKFAST	▷ TUNA, WHITE, CANNED IN OIL SOLIDS	158	23	7	0	3 OZ
10	BREAKFAST	▷ MAYONNAISE DRESSING	103	0	12	0	1 TBSP.
10	BREAKFAST	▷ BREAD, LOW CARB	60	6	2	1	1 SLICE, 1 OZ
10	BREAKFAST	▷ PICKLE RELISH, SWEET	20	0	0	5	1 TBSP.
10	BREAKFAST	▷ WATER	0	0	0	0	8 FL OZ
10	BREAKFAST	TOTAL	341	29	21	6	

DAILY SMART MEAL PLANS

Day	Meal	Food Description	Calories	Proteins	Fat	Net Carbs	Serving Size
10	BREAKFAST	TEA, BLACK, BREWED, ICED	2	0	0	1	8 FL OZ
10	*BREAKFAST*		*2*	*0*	*0*	*1*	
10	LUNCH	**HOT DOG WRAP**					
10	LUNCH	▷ FRANKFURTER, BEEF AND PORK	274	10	24	2	2 FRANK-FURTER
10	LUNCH	▷ CHEESE, COLBY	440	28	36	4	4 OZ
10	LUNCH	▷ TORTILLAS, LOW CARB, WHOLE WHEAT, FLOUR	90	3	2	3	1 TORTILLA, 28G
10	LUNCH	COFFEE, BREWED FROM GROUNDS, PREPARED WITH TAP WATER	0	0	0	0	6 FL OZ
10	LUNCH	CREAM, HEAVY	104	0	12	0	2 TBSP.
10	*LUNCH*	*TOTAL*	*908*	*41*	*74*	*9*	
10	DINNER	CORNISH GAME HENS, MEAT AND SKIN, ROASTED	660	57	45	0	9 OZ
10	DINNER	PEAS AND CARROTS, COOKED	76	4	0	12	1 CUP
10	DINNER	BUTTER, SALTED	204	0	24	0	2 TBSP.
10	DINNER	RASPBERRIES, RAW	32	1	1	4	1/2 CUP
10	DINNER	WINE, TABLE, WHITE, SAUVIGNON BLANC	119	0	0	3	5 FL OZ
10	*DINNER*	*TOTAL*	*1,091*	*62*	*70*	*19*	
11	BREAKFAST	**TORTILLA CHEESE WRAP**					
11	BREAKFAST	▷ CHEESE, MEXICAN, QUESO ASADERO	402	26	32	3	1 CUP, CUBED
11	BREAKFAST	▷ TORTILLAS, LOW CARB, WHOLE WHEAT, FLOUR	90	3	2	3	1 TORTILLA, 28G
11	BREAKFAST	▷ SALSA SAUCE, READY-TO-SERVE	38	2	0	7	1/2 CUP
11	BREAKFAST	COFFEE, BREWED FROM GROUNDS, PREPARED WITH TAP WATER	0	0	0	0	6 FL OZ
11	BREAKFAST	CREAM, HEAVY	104	0	12	0	2 TBSP.

DAILY SMART MEAL PLANS

Day	Meal	Food Description	Calories	Proteins	Fat	Net Carbs	Serving Size
11	*BREAKFAST*	*TOTAL*	*634*	*31*	*46*	*13*	
11	LUNCH	**PASTRAMI SANDWICH**					
11	LUNCH	▷ PASTRAMI	41	6	2	0	1 SLICE, 1 OZ
11	LUNCH	▷ BREAD, LOW CARB	60	6	2	1	1 SLICE, 1 OZ
11	LUNCH	**BROCCOLI WITH CHEESE**					
11	LUNCH	▷ BROCCOLI, CHOPPED, COOKED	104	12	0	8	1 CUP
11	LUNCH	▷ OIL, OLIVE, SALAD OR COOKING	115	0	13	0	1 TBSP.
11	LUNCH	▷ CHEESE, CHEDDAR	220	14	18	4	1 OZ
11	LUNCH	TEA, BLACK, BREWED, ICED	2	0	0	1	8 FL OZ
11	*LUNCH*	*TOTAL*	*542*	*38*	*35*	*14*	
11	DINNER	**HALIBUT IN WINE SAUCE**					
11	DINNER	▷ HALIBUT, ATLANTIC AND PACIFIC	188	38	2	0	6 OZ
11	DINNER	▷ CAPERS, CANNED	2	0	0	0	1 TBSP.
11	DINNER	▷ WINE, TABLE, WHITE, CHARDONNAY	62	0	0	2	2 1/2 FL OZ
11	DINNER	▷ OIL, OLIVE, SALAD OR COOKING	115	0	13	0	1 TBSP.
11	DINNER	▷ BUTTER, SALTED	102	0	12	0	1 TBSP.
11	DINNER	**ALFREDO ZUCCHINI**					
11	DINNER	▷ SQUASH, SUMMER, ALL VARIETIES, COOKED, BOILED	36	2	1	5	1 CUP
11	DINNER	▷ ALFREDO CREAM SAUCE	228	6	26	2	2 OZ
11	DINNER	COFFEE, BREWED FROM GROUNDS, PREPARED WITH TAP WATER	0	0	0	0	6 FL OZ
11	*DINNER*	*TOTAL*	*733*	*46*	*54*	*9*	
12	BREAKFAST	**GRILLED CHEESE**					

DAILY SMART MEAL PLANS

Day	Meal	Food Description	Calories	Proteins	Fat	Net Carbs	Serving Size
12	BREAKFAST	▷ CHEESE, MONTEREY	421	28	34	1	1 CUP, CUBED
12	BREAKFAST	▷ BUTTER, SALTED	104	0	24	0	2 TBSP.
12	BREAKFAST	▷ BREAD, LOW CARB	60	6	2	1	1 SLICE, 1 OZ
12	BREAKFAST	HIBISCUS TEA	0	0	0	0	8 FL OZ
12	*BREAKFAST*	*TOTAL*	*585*	*34*	*60*	*2*	
12	LUNCH	**HOT DOG WRAP**					
12	LUNCH	▷ FRANKFURTER, MEATLESS	326	27	19	6	1 CUP
12	LUNCH	▷ TORTILLAS, LOW CARB, WHOLE WHEAT, FLOUR	90	3	2	3	1 TORTILLA, 28G
12	LUNCH	**SPINACH SALAD**					
12	LUNCH	▷ SPINACH, RAW	7	1	0	0	1 CUP
12	LUNCH	▷ SALAD DRESSING, RANCH DRESSING	63	0	7	1	1 TBSP.
12	LUNCH	▷ BACON BITS, MEATLESS	33	2	2	1	1 TBSP.
12	LUNCH	▷ PECANS, DRY ROASTED	199	3	21	1	1 OZ
12	LUNCH	▷ CHEESE, FETA	75	4	6	1	1 OZ
12	LUNCH	TEA, BLACK, BREWED	2	0	0	1	6 FL OZ
12	LUNCH	CREAM, HEAVY	104	0	12	0	2 TBSP.
12	*LUNCH*	*TOTAL*	*899*	*40*	*69*	*14*	
12	DINNER	**RIBS**					
12	DINNER	▷ PORK, SPARERIBS	614	36	52	0	6 OZ
12	DINNER	▷ TERIYAKI SAUCE, READY-TO-SERVE	32	2	0	6	2 TBSP.
12	DINNER	**CAULIFLOWER WITH ALMONDS**					
12	DINNER	▷ CAULIFLOWER, COOKED	31	3	0	1	1 CUP
12	DINNER	▷ OIL, OLIVE, SALAD OR COOKING	230	0	26	0	2 TBSP.

DAILY SMART MEAL PLANS

Day	Meal	Food Description	Calories	Proteins	Fat	Net Carbs	Serving Size
12	DINNER	▷ ALMONDS, OIL ROASTED	477	17	44	6	1/2 CUP
12	DINNER	SPARKLING WATER, FLAVORED NO CALORIE	0	0	0	0	8 FL OZ
12	*DINNER*	*TOTAL*	*1,384*	*58*	*122*	*13*	
13	BREAKFAST	BAGELS, PLAIN (INCLUDES ONION, POPPY, SESAME)	72	3	0	13	1 MINI BAGEL, 2-1/2" DIA
13	BREAKFAST	CHEESE, EDAM	400	28	32	0	4 OZ
13	BREAKFAST	TOTAL	1,856	89	154	26	
13	LUNCH	**ALMOND BUTTER SANDWICH**					
13	LUNCH	▷ ALMOND BUTTER, PLAIN	98	3	9	1	1 TBSP.
13	LUNCH	▷ BREAD, LOW CARB	60	6	2	1	1 SLICE, 1 OZ
13	LUNCH	SNACKS, PORK SKINS, BARBECUE-FLAVOR	302	32	18	0	2 OZ
13	LUNCH	TEA, BLACK, BREWED, ICED	2	0	0	1	8 FL OZ
13	*LUNCH*	*TOTAL*	*462*	*41*	*29*	*3*	
13	DINNER	TURKEY BREAST, PRE-BASTED, MEAT AND SKIN, ROASTED	214	38	6	0	6 OZ
13	DINNER	**BAKED POTATO**					
13	DINNER	▷ POTATOES, BAKED, FLESH AND SKIN	57	2	0	12	1/2 CUP
13	DINNER	▷ BUTTER, SALTED	204	0	24	0	2 TBSP.
13	DINNER	▷ CREAM, SOUR, CULTURED	222	3	23	4	1/2 CUP
13	DINNER	▷ CHEESE, CHEDDAR	110	7	9	2	1 OZ
13	DINNER	CARBONATED BEVERAGE, ZERO- CALORIE, ANY FLAVOR	0	0	0	0	12 FL OZ
13	DINNER	DISTILLED, WHISKEY, 86 PROOF	105	0	0	0	1 JIGGER, 1/2 FL OZ
13	*DINNER*	*TOTAL*	*912*	*50*	*62*	*18*	

DAILY SMART MEAL PLANS

Day	Meal	Food Description	Calories	Proteins	Fat	Net Carbs	Serving Size
14	BREAKFAST	**TORTILLA CHEESE WRAP**					
14	BREAKFAST	▷ CHEESE, CHEDDAR	330	21	27	6	3 OZ
14	BREAKFAST	▷ TORTILLAS, LOW CARB, WHOLE WHEAT, FLOUR	90	3	2	3	1 TORTILLA, 28G
14	BREAKFAST	TEA, BLACK, BREWED	2	0	0	1	6 FL OZ
14	BREAKFAST	CREAM, HEAVY	104	0	12	0	2 TBSP.
14	*BREAKFAST*	*TOTAL*	*526*	*24*	*41*	*10*	
14	LUNCH	**HAM WRAP**					
14	LUNCH	▷ HAM WITH NATURAL JUICES, PAN-BROIL	153	22	7	0	3 OZ
14	LUNCH	▷ LETTUCE, BUTTERHEAD (INCLUDES BOSTON AND BIBB TYPES), RAW	7	1	0	0	1 CUP
14	LUNCH	▷ CHEESE, SWISS	502	36	37	7	1 CUP, CUBED
14	LUNCH	WATER	0	0	0	0	8 FL OZ
14	*LUNCH*	*TOTAL*	*662*	*59*	*44*	*7*	
14	DINNER	PORK, BACK RIBS, ROASTED	496	40	36	0	6 OZ
14	DINNER	STEAK SAUCE, TOMATO BASED	32	0	0	6	2 TBSP.
14	DINNER	**SALAD**					
14	DINNER	▷ LETTUCE, COS OR ROMAINE, RAW	8	1	0	1	1 CUP
14	DINNER	▷ MUSHROOMS, OYSTER, RAW	5	0	0	1	1 SMALL
14	DINNER	▷ CUCUMBER, WITH PEEL, RAW	8	0	0	2	1/2 CUP
14	DINNER	▷ CARROTS, BABY, RAW	4	0	0	1	1 MEDIUM
14	DINNER	▷ TOMATOES, RED, RAW	16	1	0	3	1/2 CUP
14	DINNER	▷ BROCCOLI, FLOWER CLUSTERS, RAW	10	1	0	2	1/2 CUP
14	DINNER	▷ CREAMY DRESSING, MADE WITH SOUR CREAM AND/OR BUTTERMILK AND OIL, REDUCED CALORIE	48	0	4	2	2 TBSP.

DAILY SMART MEAL PLANS

Day	Meal	Food Description	Calories	Proteins	Fat	Net Carbs	Serving Size
14	DINNER	SPARKLING WATER	0	0	0	0	8 FL OZ
14	*DINNER*	*TOTAL*	*627*	*43*	*40*	*18*	

WEEK THREE

Day	Meal	Food Description	Calories	Proteins	Fat	Net Carbs	Serving Size
15	BREAKFAST	**SAUSAGE WRAP**					
15	BREAKFAST	▷ SAUSAGE, CHICKEN AND BEEF, SMOKED	407	26	33	0	1 CUP
15	BREAKFAST	▷ TORTILLAS, LOW CARB, WHOLE WHEAT, FLOUR	90	3	2	3	1 TORTILLA, 28G
15	BREAKFAST	WATER	0	0	0	0	8 FL OZ
15	*BREAKFAST*	*TOTAL*	*497*	*29*	*35*	*3*	
15	LUNCH	POLISH SAUSAGE, PORK	554	24	48	2	6 OZ
15	LUNCH	CHEESE, MONTEREY	211	14	17	1	4 OZ
15	LUNCH	**RASPBERRIES AND CREAM**					
15	LUNCH	▷ RASPBERRIES, RAW	64	1	1	7	1 CUP
15	LUNCH	▷ CREAM, HEAVY	104	0	12	0	2 TBSP.
15	LUNCH	HIBISCUS TEA	0	0	0	0	8 FL OZ
15	*LUNCH*	*TOTAL*	*933*	*39*	*78*	*10*	
15	DINNER	BEEF, SHORT LOIN, PORTERHOUSE STEAK	470	44	32	0	6 OZ
15	DINNER	CORN, SWEET, YELLOW, FROZEN, BOILED	65	2	1	13	1/2 CUP
15	DINNER	BUTTER, SALTED	204	0	24	0	2 TBSP.
15	DINNER	TEA, BLACK, BREWED	2	0	0	1	6 FL OZ
15	DINNER	CREAM, HEAVY	104	0	12	0	2 TBSP.
15	*DINNER*	*TOTAL*	*845*	*46*	*69*	*14*	
16	BREAKFAST	**BURGER WRAP**					
16	BREAKFAST	▷ BEEF, GROUND, 70% LEAN MEAT / 30% FAT	422	40	28	0	6 OZ

DAILY SMART MEAL PLANS

Day	Meal	Food Description	Calories	Proteins	Fat	Net Carbs	Serving Size
16	BREAKFAST	▷ LETTUCE, BUTTERHEAD (INCLUDES BOSTON AND BIBB TYPES), RAW	7	1	0	0	1 CUP
16	BREAKFAST	▷ CATSUP	17	0	0	5	1 TBSP.
16	BREAKFAST	WATER	0	0	0	0	8 FL OZ
16	*BREAKFAST*	*TOTAL*	*446*	*41*	*28*	*5*	
16	LUNCH	**ITALIAN SAUSAGE SANDWICH**					
16	LUNCH	▷ SAUSAGE, ITALIAN, SWEET, LINKS	125	14	7	2	1 LINK, 3 OZ
16	LUNCH	▷ CHEESE, MOZZARELLA, WHOLE MILK	170	12	12	2	2 OZ
16	LUNCH	▷ BREAD, LOW CARB	60	6	2	1	1 SLICE, 1 OZ
16	LUNCH	▷ OLIVES, RIPE, CANNED	46	0	4	2	2 OZ
16	LUNCH	TEA, BLACK, BREWED, ICED	2	0	0	1	8 FL OZ
16	*LUNCH*	*TOTAL*	*403*	*32*	*25*	*8*	
16	DINNER	SAUSAGE, ITALIAN, SWEET, LINKS	375	42	21	6	3 LINKS, 3 OZ
16	DINNER	PASTA SAUCE, MARINARA, READY-TO-SERVE	160	2	14	6	1 CUP
16	DINNER	SQUASH, SUMMER, ALL VARIETIES, COOKED, BOILED	36	2	1	5	1 CUP
16	DINNER	BUTTER, SALTED	204	0	24	0	2 TBSP.
16	DINNER	SPARKLING WATER	0	0	0	0	8 FL OZ
16	*DINNER*	*TOTAL*	*775*	*46*	*60*	*17*	
17	BREAKFAST	**CHORIZO WRAP**					
17	BREAKFAST	▷ CHORIZO, PORK AND BEEF	254	14	22	2	2 OZ
17	BREAKFAST	▷ EGG, WHOLE, COOKED, SCRAMBLED	188	12	12	0	4 OZ
17	BREAKFAST	▷ ONIONS, COOKED	14	0	0	4	2 TBSP.
17	BREAKFAST	TEA, BLACK, BREWED, ICED	2	0	0	1	8 FL OZ
17	*BREAKFAST*	*TOTAL*	*458*	*26*	*34*	*7*	

DAILY SMART MEAL PLANS

Day	Meal	Food Description	Calories	Proteins	Fat	Net Carbs	Serving Size
17	LUNCH	**TURKEY WRAP**					
17	LUNCH	▷ GROUND TURKEY, 85% LEAN, 15% FAT	219	21	15	0	3 OZ
17	LUNCH	▷ CHEESE, MOZZARELLA, WHOLE MILK	85	6	6	1	1 OZ
17	LUNCH	▷ TORTILLAS, LOW CARB, WHOLE WHEAT, FLOUR	90	3	2	3	1 TORTILLA, 28G
17	LUNCH	COFFEE, BREWED FROM GROUNDS, PREPARED WITH TAP WATER	0	0	0	0	6 FL OZ
17	LUNCH	CREAM, HEAVY	104	0	12	0	2 TBSP.
17	*LUNCH*	*TOTAL*	*498*	*30*	*35*	*4*	
17	DINNER	**TEMPEH STIR-FRY**					
17	DINNER	▷ TEMPEH	346	34	12	6	6 OZ
17	DINNER	▷ PEPPERS, SWEET, RED, COOKED	19	1	0	4	1/2 CUP
17	DINNER	▷ ONIONS, YELLOW, SAUTÉED	58	1	5	3	1/2 CUP
17	DINNER	▷ BROCCOLI, CHOPPED, COOKED	52	6	0	4	1 CUP
17	DINNER	▷ MUSHROOMS, WHITE, RAW	21	3	0	2	1 CUP
17	DINNER	▷ SOY SAUCE MADE FROM SOY (TAMARI)	22	4	0	2	2 TBSP.
17	DINNER	▷ OIL, OLIVE, SALAD OR COOKING	230	0	26	0	2 TBSP.
17	DINNER	TEA, INSTANT, UNSWEETENED	0	0	0	0	1 TSP
17	*DINNER*	*TOTAL*	*748*	*49*	*43*	*21*	
18	BREAKFAST	PORK SAUSAGE, LINK/PATTY, FULLY MICROWAVED	368	12	36	0	4 LINKS
18	BREAKFAST	CHEESE, MONTEREY	211	14	17	1	1/2 CUP, CUBED
18	BREAKFAST	CARROTS, RAW	52	1	0	8	1 CUP
18	BREAKFAST	COFFEE, BREWED FROM GROUNDS, PREPARED WITH TAP WATER	0	0	0	0	6 FL OZ

DAILY SMART MEAL PLANS

Day	Meal	Food Description	Calories	Proteins	Fat	Net Carbs	Serving Size
18	BREAKFAST	CREAM, HEAVY	104	0	12	0	2 TBSP.
18	BREAKFAST	TOTAL	735	27	65	9	
18	LUNCH	**TURKEY WRAP**					
18	LUNCH	▷ TURKEY, BREAST, MEAT AND SKIN, ROASTED	278	50	10	0	6 OZ
18	LUNCH	▷ LETTUCE, BUTTERHEAD (INCLUDES BOSTON AND BIBB TYPES), RAW	7	1	0	0	1 CUP
18	LUNCH	▷ CHEESE, PASTEURIZED PROCESS, AMERICAN	204	10	18	2	2 OZ
18	LUNCH	WATER	0	0	0	0	8 FL OZ
18	LUNCH	TOTAL	489	61	28	2	
18	DINNER	**ROAST BEEF SANDWICH**					
18	DINNER	▷ ROAST BEEF, DELI STYLE, PREPACKAGED, SLICED	60	12	0	0	6 SLICE, OVAL
18	DINNER	▷ LETTUCE, BUTTERHEAD (INCLUDES BOSTON AND BIBB TYPES), RAW	7	1	0	0	1 CUP
18	DINNER	▷ HORSERADISH, PREPARED	7	0	0	2	1 TBSP.
18	DINNER	▷ MAYONNAISE DRESSING	103	0	12	0	1 TBSP.
18	DINNER	▷ BREAD, LOW CARB	120	12	4	2	2 SLICE, 1 OZ
18	DINNER	SNACKS, PORK SKINS, BARBECUE-FLAVOR	151	16	9	0	1 OZ
18	DINNER	CREAM, SOUR, CULTURED	444	5	45	7	1 CUP
18	DINNER	COFFEE, BREWED FROM GROUNDS, PREPARED WITH TAP WATER	0	0	0	0	6 FL OZ
18	DINNER	CREAM, HEAVY	104	0	12	0	2 TBSP.
18	DINNER	TOTAL	996	46	82	11	
19	BREAKFAST	EGG, WHOLE, COOKED, HARD-BOILED	308	24	20	4	4 LARGE
19	BREAKFAST	BUTTER, SALTED	104	0	24	0	2 TBSP.

DAILY SMART MEAL PLANS

Day	Meal	Food Description	Calories	Proteins	Fat	Net Carbs	Serving Size
19	BREAKFAST	BREAD, LOW CARB	60	6	2	1	1 SLICE, 1 OZ
19	BREAKFAST	HIBISCUS TEA	0	0	0	0	8 FL OZ
19	*BREAKFAST*	*TOTAL*	*472*	*30*	*46*	*5*	
19	LUNCH	**CHORIZO WRAP**					
19	LUNCH	▷ CHORIZO, PORK AND BEEF	254	14	22	2	2 OZ
19	LUNCH	▷ CHEESE, MEXICAN, QUESO ASADERO	201	13	16	2	1/2 CUP, CUBED
19	LUNCH	▷ SALSA SAUCE, VERDE, READY-TO-SERVE	11	0	0	1	2 TBSP.
19	LUNCH	▷ TORTILLAS, LOW CARB, WHOLE WHEAT, FLOUR	90	3	2	3	1 TORTILLA, 28G
19	LUNCH	TEA, BLACK, BREWED	2	0	0	1	6 FL OZ
19	LUNCH	CREAM, HEAVY	104	0	12	0	2 TBSP.
19	*LUNCH*	*TOTAL*	*662*	*30*	*52*	*9*	
19	DINNER	**CHICKEN WRAP**					
19	DINNER	▷ CHICKEN, BROILER, ROTISSERIE, GRILLED, BREAST MEAT AND SKIN	149	22	7	0	3 OZ
19	DINNER	▷ SALSA SAUCE, READY-TO-SERVE	38	2	0	7	1/2 CUP
19	DINNER	▷ CHEESE, MEXICAN, QUESO QUESADILLA	400	28	32	0	4 OZ
19	DINNER	▷ TOMATOES, RED, RAW	16	1	0	3	1/2 CUP
19	DINNER	▷ TORTILLAS, LOW CARB, WHOLE WHEAT, FLOUR	180	6	4	6	2 TORTILLAS, 28G
19	DINNER	SPARKLING WATER	0	0	0	0	8 FL OZ
19	*DINNER*	*TOTAL*	*783*	*59*	*43*	*16*	
20	BREAKFAST	**FRIED EGG SANDWICH**					
20	BREAKFAST	▷ EGG, WHOLE, COOKED, FRIED	360	24	28	0	4 LARGE
20	BREAKFAST	▷ OIL, OLIVE, SALAD OR COOKING	115	0	13	0	1 TBSP.

DAILY SMART MEAL PLANS

Day	Meal	Food Description	Calories	Proteins	Fat	Net Carbs	Serving Size
20	BREAKFAST	▷ BREAD, LOW CARB	60	6	2	1	1 SLICE, 1 OZ
20	BREAKFAST	TEA, BLACK, BREWED	2	0	0	1	6 FL OZ
20	BREAKFAST	CREAM, HEAVY	104	0	12	0	2 TBSP.
20	BREAKFAST	TOTAL	641	30	55	2	
20	BREAKFAST	CHEESE, MEXICAN, QUESO QUESADILLA	200	14	16	0	2 OZ
		Total	200	14	16	0	
20	LUNCH	**ROAST BEEF WRAP**					
20	LUNCH	▷ ROAST BEEF, DELI STYLE, PREPACKAGED, SLICED	10	2	0	0	1 SLICE, OVAL
20	LUNCH	▷ HORSERADISH, PREPARED	7	0	0	2	1 TBSP.
20	LUNCH	▷ TORTILLAS, LOW CARB, WHOLE WHEAT, FLOUR	90	3	2	3	1 TORTILLA, 28G
20	LUNCH	**KALE SALAD**					
20	LUNCH	▷ KALE, RAW	16	2	0	0	2 CUP
20	LUNCH	▷ SALAD DRESSING, BACON AND TOMATO	49	0	5	0	1 TBSP.
20	LUNCH	▷ EGG, WHOLE, COOKED, HARD-BOILED	211	17	14	2	1 CUP
20	LUNCH	▷ SUNFLOWER SEED KERNELS, OIL ROASTED	168	6	15	3	1 OZ
20	LUNCH	WATER	0	0	0	0	8 FL OZ
20	LUNCH	TOTAL	551	30	36	10	
20	DINNER	PORK, LOIN, TENDERLOIN	342	50	14	0	6 OZ
20	DINNER	BUTTER, SALTED	204	0	24	0	2 TBSP.
20	DINNER	CARROTS, COOKED	27	1	0	4	1/2 CUP
20	DINNER	BUTTER, SALTED	204	0	24	0	2 TBSP.
20	DINNER	SPARKLING WATER	0	0	0	0	8 FL OZ
20	DINNER	TOTAL	777	51	62	4	

DAILY SMART MEAL PLANS

Day	Meal	Food Description	Calories	Proteins	Fat	Net Carbs	Serving Size
21	BREAKFAST	EGG, WHOLE, COOKED, POACHED	288	24	20	0	4 LARGE
21	BREAKFAST	BUTTER, SALTED	104	0	24	0	2 TBSP.
21	BREAKFAST	BREAD, LOW CARB	60	6	2	1	1 SLICE, 1 OZ
21	BREAKFAST	WATER	0	0	0	0	8 FL OZ
21	*BREAKFAST*	*TOTAL*	*452*	*30*	*46*	*1*	
21	LUNCH	**SALAMI SANDWICH**					
21	LUNCH	▷ SALAMI, DRY OR HARD, PORK, BEEF	424	24	36	0	4 OZ
21	LUNCH	▷ CHEESE, PROVOLONE	200	14	16	2	2 OZ
21	LUNCH	▷ BREAD, LOW CARB	60	6	2	1	1 SLICE, 1 OZ
21	LUNCH	ICED COFFEE, BREWED FROM GROUNDS, PREPARED WITH TAP WATER	0	0	0	0	6 FL OZ
21	*LUNCH*	*TOTAL*	*684*	*44*	*54*	*3*	
21	DINNER	SCALLOP (BAY AND SEA), STEAMED	188	34	2	10	6 OZ
21	DINNER	BUTTER, SALTED	204	0	24	0	2 TBSP.
21	DINNER	**SAUTÉED VEGGIES AND CHEESE**					
21	DINNER	▷ SQUASH, SUMMER, ALL VARIETIES, COOKED, BOILED	18	1	1	3	1/2 CUP
21	DINNER	▷ PEPPERS, SWEET, RED, COOKED	19	1	0	4	1/2 CUP
21	DINNER	▷ BROCCOLI, CHOPPED, COOKED	26	3	0	2	1/2 CUP
21	DINNER	▷ GARLIC, RAW	4	0	0	1	1 TSP
21	DINNER	▷ CHEESE, PARMESAN, HARD	110	10	7	1	1 OZ
21	DINNER	▷ BUTTER, SALTED	204	0	24	0	2 TBSP.
21	DINNER	SPARKLING WATER	0	0	0	0	8 FL OZ
21	*DINNER*	*TOTAL*	*773*	*49*	*58*	*21*	

DAILY SMART MEAL PLANS

Day	Meal	Food Description	Calories	Proteins	Fat	Net Carbs	Serving Size
WEEK FOUR							
22	BREAKFAST	**SCRAMBLED EGG SANDWICH**					
22	BREAKFAST	▷ EGG, WHOLE, COOKED, OMELET	352	24	24	0	8 OZ
22	BREAKFAST	▷ BUTTER, SALTED	104	0	24	0	2 TBSP.
22	BREAKFAST	▷ BREAD, LOW CARB	60	6	2	1	1 SLICE, 1 OZ
22	BREAKFAST	TEA, BLACK, BREWED, ICED	2	0	0	1	8 FL OZ
22	*BREAKFAST*	*TOTAL*	*518*	*30*	*50*	*2*	
22	LUNCH	SAUSAGE, SUMMER, PORK AND BEEF, STICKS, WITH CHEDDAR CHEESE	476	20	44	4	4 OZ
22	LUNCH	CHEESE, GRUYERE	232	16	18	0	2 OZ
22	LUNCH	TEA, BLACK, BREWED, ICED	2	0	0	1	8 FL OZ
22	*LUNCH*	*TOTAL*	*710*	*36*	*62*	*5*	
22	DINNER	SAUSAGE, SMOKED LINK SAUSAGE, PORK AND BEEF	544	20	48	4	6 OZ
22	DINNER	**SALAD**					
22	DINNER	▷ LETTUCE, BUTTERHEAD (INCLUDES BOSTON AND BIBB TYPES), RAW	7	1	0	0	1 CUP
22	DINNER	▷ TOMATOES, RED CHERRY, RAW	27	1	0	4	1 CUP
22	DINNER	▷ SQUASH, SUMMER, ALL VARIETIES, RAW	9	1	0	2	1/2 CUP
22	DINNER	▷ ALMONDS, OIL ROASTED	477	17	44	6	1/2 CUP
22	DINNER	▷ SALAD DRESSING, ITALIAN DRESSING	82	0	8	2	2 TBSP.
22	DINNER	TEA, BLACK, BREWED	2	0	0	1	6 FL OZ
22	DINNER	CREAM, HEAVY	104	0	12	0	2 TBSP.
22	*DINNER*	*TOTAL*	*1,252*	*40*	*112*	*19*	

DAILY SMART MEAL PLANS

Day	Meal	Food Description	Calories	Proteins	Fat	Net Carbs	Serving Size
23	BREAKFAST	EGG, WHOLE, COOKED, SCRAMBLED	376	24	24	0	8 OZ
23	BREAKFAST	BUTTER, SALTED	104	0	24	0	2 TBSP.
23	BREAKFAST	BREAD, LOW CARB	60	6	2	1	1 SLICE, 1 OZ
23	BREAKFAST	COFFEE, BREWED FROM GROUNDS, PREPARED WITH TAP WATER	0	0	0	0	6 FL OZ
23	BREAKFAST	CREAM, HEAVY	104	0	12	0	2 TBSP.
23	*BREAKFAST*	*TOTAL*	*644*	*30*	*62*	*1*	
23	LUNCH	**TURKEY WRAP**					
23	LUNCH	▷ TURKEY BREAST, PRE-BASTED, MEAT AND SKIN, ROASTED	214	38	6	0	6 OZ
23	LUNCH	▷ CHEESE, CREAM	96	2	10	2	2 TBSP.
23	LUNCH	▷ AVOCADOS, RAW, CALIFORNIA	192	3	18	2	1/2 CUP
23	LUNCH	▷ LETTUCE, BUTTERHEAD (INCLUDES BOSTON AND BIBB TYPES), RAW	7	1	0	0	1 CUP
23	LUNCH	HIBISCUS TEA	0	0	0	0	8 FL OZ
23	*LUNCH*	*TOTAL*	*509*	*44*	*34*	*4*	
23	DINNER	**CHORIZO WRAP**					
23	DINNER	▷ CHORIZO, PORK AND BEEF	508	28	44	4	4 OZ
23	DINNER	▷ SALSA SAUCE, READY-TO-SERVE	38	2	0	7	1/2 CUP
23	DINNER	▷ CHEESE, MEXICAN, QUESO QUESADILLA	400	28	32	0	4 OZ
23	DINNER	▷ TOMATOES, RED, RAW	16	1	0	3	1/2 CUP
23	DINNER	▷ TORTILLAS, LOW CARB, WHOLE WHEAT, FLOUR	180	6	4	6	2 TORTILLAS, 28G
23	DINNER	SPARKLING WATER	0	0	0	0	8 FL OZ
23	*DINNER*	*TOTAL*	*1,142*	*65*	*80*	*20*	

DAILY SMART MEAL PLANS

Day	Meal	Food Description	Calories	Proteins	Fat	Net Carbs	Serving Size
24	BREAKFAST	PEPPERONI, PORK, BEEF	276	12	24	0	2 OZ
24	BREAKFAST	CHEESE, CHEDDAR	330	21	27	6	3 OZ
24	BREAKFAST	HIBISCUS TEA	0	0	0	0	8 FL OZ
24	*BREAKFAST*	*TOTAL*	*606*	*33*	*51*	*6*	
24	LUNCH	**BACON AND EGG SANDWICH**					
24	LUNCH	▷ BACON, PAN-FRIED, BROILED OR ROASTED	172	12	12	0	4 SLICES
24	LUNCH	▷ EGG, WHOLE, COOKED, SCRAMBLED	80	4	8	0	4 TBSP.
24	LUNCH	▷ CHEESE, COLBY	110	7	9	1	1 OZ
24	LUNCH	▷ TOMATOES, RED, RAW	16	1	0	3	1/2 CUP
24	LUNCH	▷ LETTUCE, GREEN LEAF, RAW	5	0	0	1	1 CUP
24	LUNCH	▷ MAYONNAISE DRESSING	206	0	24	0	2 TBSP.
24	LUNCH	▷ BREAD, LOW CARB	120	12	4	2	2 SLICE, 1 OZ
24	LUNCH	BLACKBERRIES, RAW	31	1	1	3	1/2 CUP
24	LUNCH	TEA, BLACK, BREWED, ICED	2	0	0	1	8 FL OZ
24	*LUNCH*	*TOTAL*	*742*	*37*	*58*	*11*	
24	DINNER	**CHICKEN STIR-FRY**					
24	DINNER	▷ CHICKEN, BROILER, BREAST MEAT ONLY	244	48	6	0	6 OZ
24	DINNER	▷ MUSHROOMS, WHITE, COOKED	44	3	1	5	1 CUP
24	DINNER	▷ ONIONS, COOKED	14	0	0	4	2 TBSP.
24	DINNER	▷ SQUASH, SUMMER, ALL VARIETIES, COOKED, BOILED	9	1	0	2	1/2 CUP
24	DINNER	▷ BAMBOO SHOOTS, CANNED, DRAINED SOLIDS	25	2	1	2	1 CUP
24	DINNER	▷ OYSTER SAUCE, READY-TO-SERVE	9	0	0	2	1 TBSP.

DAILY SMART MEAL PLANS

Day	Meal	Food Description	Calories	Proteins	Fat	Net Carbs	Serving Size
24	DINNER	▷ SOY SAUCE MADE FROM SOY (TAMARI)	11	2	0	1	1 TBSP.
24	DINNER	▷ OIL, CORN, PEANUT, AND OLIVE	248	0	28	0	2 TBSP.
24	DINNER	TEA, BLACK, BREWED, ICED	2	0	0	1	8 FL OZ
24	*DINNER*	*TOTAL*	*606*	*56*	*36*	*17*	
25	BREAKFAST	**TURKEY WRAP**					
25	BREAKFAST	▷ TURKEY BREAST, LUNCHEON MEAT	128	24	0	4	4 SLICES
25	BREAKFAST	▷ LETTUCE, BUTTERHEAD (INCLUDES BOSTON AND BIBB TYPES), RAW	7	1	0	0	1 CUP
25	BREAKFAST	▷ SALAD DRESSING, CAESAR DRESSING	76	0	8	0	1 TBSP.
25	BREAKFAST	WATER	0	0	0	0	8 FL OZ
25	*BREAKFAST*	*TOTAL*	*211*	*25*	*8*	*4*	
25	LUNCH	**TURKEY WRAP**					
25	LUNCH	▷ TURKEY BREAST, SLICED, OVEN ROASTED, LUNCHEON MEAT	88	16	0	4	4 SLICES
25	LUNCH	▷ LETTUCE, RED LEAF, RAW	4	0	0	1	1 CUP
25	LUNCH	▷ AVOCADOS, RAW, CALIFORNIA	192	3	18	2	1/2 CUP
25	LUNCH	▷ CHEESE, MOZZARELLA, WHOLE MILK	340	24	24	4	4 OZ
25	LUNCH	▷ SALAD DRESSING, FRENCH DRESSING	73	0	7	2	1 TBSP.
25	LUNCH	WATER	0	0	0	0	8 FL OZ
25	*LUNCH*	*TOTAL*	*697*	*43*	*49*	*13*	
25	DINNER	**BURGER SANDWICH**					
25	DINNER	▷ BEEF, GROUND, 70% LEAN MEAT / 30% FAT	422	40	28	0	6 OZ
25	DINNER	▷ LETTUCE, BUTTERHEAD (INCLUDES BOSTON AND BIBB TYPES), RAW	7	1	0	0	1 CUP

DAILY SMART MEAL PLANS

Day	Meal	Food Description	Calories	Proteins	Fat	Net Carbs	Serving Size
25	DINNER	▷ MAYONNAISE DRESSING	103	0	12	0	1 TBSP.
25	DINNER	▷ CATSUP	17	0	0	5	1 TBSP.
25	DINNER	▷ BACON, PAN-FRIED, MICROWAVED OR ROASTED	86	6	6	0	2 SLICES
25	DINNER	▷ AVOCADOS, RAW, CALIFORNIA	192	3	18	2	1/2 CUP
25	DINNER	▷ BREAD, LOW CARB	120	12	4	2	2 SLICE, 1 OZ
25	DINNER	APPLES, RAW, WITH SKIN	62	0	0	12	1 CUP
25	DINNER	COFFEE, BREWED FROM GROUNDS, PREPARED WITH TAP WATER	0	0	0	0	6 FL OZ
25	DINNER	CREAM, HEAVY	104	0	12	0	2 TBSP.
25	*DINNER*	*TOTAL*	*1,113*	*62*	*80*	*21*	
26	BREAKFAST	**BACON WRAP**					
26	BREAKFAST	▷ BACON, PAN-FRIED, BROILED OR ROASTED	172	12	12	0	4 SLICES
26	BREAKFAST	▷ MAYONNAISE DRESSING	103	0	12	0	1 TBSP.
26	BREAKFAST	▷ LETTUCE, BUTTERHEAD (INCLUDES BOSTON AND BIBB TYPES), RAW	7	1	0	0	1 CUP
26	BREAKFAST	▷ CHEESE, COLBY	220	14	18	2	2 OZ
26	BREAKFAST	▷ TORTILLAS, LOW CARB, WHOLE WHEAT, FLOUR	90	3	2	3	1 TORTILLA, 28G
26	BREAKFAST	WATER	0	0	0	0	8 FL OZ
26	*BREAKFAST*	*TOTAL*	*592*	*30*	*44*	*5*	
26	LUNCH	PEPPERONI, PORK, BEEF	414	18	36	0	3 OZ
26	LUNCH	CHEESE, MOZZARELLA, WHOLE MILK	170	12	12	2	2 OZ
26	LUNCH	WATER	0	0	0	0	8 FL OZ
26	*LUNCH*	*TOTAL*	*584*	*30*	*48*	*2*	

DAILY SMART MEAL PLANS

Day	Meal	Food Description	Calories	Proteins	Fat	Net Carbs	Serving Size
26	DINNER	**WINGS**					
26	DINNER	▷ CHICKEN, ROTISSERIE, WING MEAT AND SKIN	524	48	36	0	4 WINGS
26	DINNER	▷ WING HOT SAUCE, READY-TO-SERVE	120	0	12	4	4 TBSP.
26	DINNER	CELERY, RAW	16	1	0	1	1 CUP
26	DINNER	CARROTS, RAW	52	1	0	8	1 CUP
26	DINNER	SALAD DRESSING, BLUE OR ROQUEFORT CHEESE DRESSING	292	0	32	4	4 TBSP.
26	DINNER	SPARKLING WATER	0	0	0	0	8 FL OZ
26	*DINNER*	*TOTAL*	*1,004*	*50*	*80*	*17*	
27	BREAKFAST	**TURKEY BACON SANDWICH**					
27	BREAKFAST	▷ TURKEY BACON, MICROWAVED	116	8	8	0	4 SLICES
27	BREAKFAST	▷ LETTUCE, BUTTERHEAD (INCLUDES BOSTON AND BIBB TYPES), RAW	7	1	0	0	1 CUP
27	BREAKFAST	▷ CHEESE, CHEDDAR	220	14	18	4	2 OZ
27	BREAKFAST	▷ BUTTER, SALTED	104	0	24	0	2 TBSP.
27	BREAKFAST	▷ BREAD, LOW CARB	60	6	2	1	1 SLICE, 1 OZ
27	BREAKFAST	WATER	0	0	0	0	8 FL OZ
27	*BREAKFAST*	*TOTAL*	*507*	*29*	*52*	*5*	
27	LUNCH	**KIELBASA, POLISH, TURKEY AND BEEF, SMOKED**	254	14	20	4	4 OZ
27	LUNCH	▷ AVOCADOS, RAW, CALIFORNIA	384	5	35	4	1 CUP
27	LUNCH	▷ LETTUCE, BUTTERHEAD (INCLUDES BOSTON AND BIBB TYPES), RAW	7	1	0	0	1 CUP
27	LUNCH	▷ CHEESE, MUENSTER	208	13	17	1	1/2 CUP
27	LUNCH	TEA, BLACK, BREWED	2	0	0	1	6 FL OZ

DAILY SMART MEAL PLANS

Day	Meal	Food Description	Calories	Proteins	Fat	Net Carbs	Serving Size
27	LUNCH	CREAM, HEAVY	104	0	12	0	2 TBSP.
27	*LUNCH*	*TOTAL*	*959*	*33*	*84*	*10*	
27	LUNCH	SALAD					
27	DINNER	SHRIMP, MIXED SPECIES	44	10	0	0	8 LG
27	DINNER	SHRIMP COCKTAIL SAUCE, READY-TO-SERVE	30	0	0	8	2 TBSP.
27	DINNER	**SALAD**					
27	DINNER	▷ LETTUCE, RED LEAF, RAW	4	0	0	1	1 CUP
27	DINNER	▷ AVOCADOS, RAW, CALIFORNIA	384	5	35	4	1 CUP
27	DINNER	▷ CHEESE, PARMESAN, GRATED	242	22	16	2	2 OZ
27	DINNER	▷ MUSHROOMS, WHITE, RAW	21	3	0	2	1 CUP
27	DINNER	▷ SALAD DRESSING, SESAME SEED DRESSING	132	0	14	2	2 TBSP.
27	DINNER	SPARKLING WATER	0	0	0	0	8 FL OZ
27	*DINNER*	*TOTAL*	*857*	*40*	*65*	*19*	
		WEEK FIVE					
28	BREAKFAST	**CANADIAN BACON WRAP**					
28	BREAKFAST	▷ CANADIAN BACON, PAN-FRIED	261	33	12	3	4 SLICES
28	BREAKFAST	▷ BUTTER, SALTED	104	0	24	0	2 TBSP.
28	BREAKFAST	▷ TORTILLAS, LOW CARB, WHOLE WHEAT, FLOUR	90	3	2	3	1 TORTILLA, 28G
28	BREAKFAST	TEA, BLACK, BREWED	2	0	0	1	6 FL OZ
28	BREAKFAST	CREAM, HEAVY	104	0	12	0	2 TBSP.
28	*BREAKFAST*	*TOTAL*	*561*	*36*	*50*	*7*	

DAILY SMART MEAL PLANS

Day	Meal	Food Description	Calories	Proteins	Fat	Net Carbs	Serving Size
28	LUNCH	**PEANUT BUTTER SANDWICH**					
28	LUNCH	▷ PEANUT BUTTER, SMOOTH STYLE	382	14	32	10	2 TBSP.
28	LUNCH	▷ BREAD, LOW CARB	60	6	2	1	1 SLICE, 1 OZ
28	LUNCH	CHEESE, GRUYERE	232	16	18	0	2 OZ
28	LUNCH	TEA, BLACK, BREWED, ICED	2	0	0	1	8 FL OZ
28	*LUNCH*	*TOTAL*	*676*	*36*	*52*	*12*	
28	DINNER	**BAKED MEATBALLS**					
28	DINNER	▷ MEATBALLS, FROZEN, ITALIAN STYLE	486	24	38	10	6 OZ
28	DINNER	▷ PASTA SAUCE, MARINARA, READY-TO-SERVE	80	1	7	3	1/2 CUP
28	DINNER	▷ CHEESE, MOZZARELLA, WHOLE MILK	340	24	24	4	4 OZ
28	DINNER	WINE, TABLE, RED, PINOT NOIR	121	0	0	3	5 FL OZ
28	*DINNER*	*TOTAL*	*1,027*	*49*	*69*	*20*	

WEEK FIVE

Day	Meal	Food Description	Calories	Proteins	Fat	Net Carbs	Serving Size
29	BREAKFAST	BACON AND BEEF STICKS	290	16	24	0	2 OZ
29	BREAKFAST	CHEESE, GRUYERE	232	16	18	0	2 OZ
29	BREAKFAST	TEA, BLACK, BREWED, ICED	2	0	0	1	8 FL OZ
29	*BREAKFAST*	*TOTAL*	*524*	*32*	*42*	*1*	
29	LUNCH	TROUT, RAINBOW, FARMED	286	40	12	0	6 OZ
29	LUNCH	OIL, OLIVE, SALAD OR COOKING	230	0	26	0	2 TBSP.
29	LUNCH	ASPARAGUS, COOKED	32	5	1	0	1 CUP
29	LUNCH	CHEESE, PARMESAN, SHREDDED	42	4	2	0	2 TBSP.
29	LUNCH	BUTTER, SALTED	102	0	12	0	1 TBSP.

DAILY SMART MEAL PLANS

Day	Meal	Food Description	Calories	Proteins	Fat	Net Carbs	Serving Size
29	LUNCH	COFFEE, BREWED FROM GROUNDS, PREPARED WITH TAP WATER	0	0	0	0	6 FL OZ
29	LUNCH	CREAM, HEAVY	104	0	12	0	2 TBSP.
29	*LUNCH*	*TOTAL*	*796*	*49*	*65*	*0*	
29	DINNER	**OMELET**					
29	DINNER	▷ 4 MEDIUM EGGS, WHOLE, COOKED, OMELET	320	22	14	0	1 SERVING
29	DINNER	▷ CHEESE, CHEDDAR	220	14	18	4	2 OZ
29	DINNER	▷ AVOCADOS, RAW, CALIFORNIA	192	3	18	2	1/2 CUP
29	DINNER	▷ BROCCOLI, FLOWER CLUSTERS, RAW	10	1	0	2	1/2 CUP
29	DINNER	▷ ONIONS, COOKED	14	0	0	4	2 TBSP.
29	DINNER	▷ BUTTER, SALTED	204	0	24	0	2 TBSP.
29	DINNER	TEA, BLACK, BREWED	2	0	0	1	6 FL OZ
29	DINNER	CREAM, HEAVY	104	0	12	0	2 TBSP.
29	*DINNER*	*TOTAL*	*1,066*	*40*	*86*	*13*	
30	BREAKFAST	PEANUT BUTTER, CHUNK STYLE	188	8	16	4	2 TBSP.
30	BREAKFAST	CRACKERS, LOW CARB	100	4	7	6	10 CRACKERS
30	BREAKFAST	COFFEE, BREWED FROM GROUNDS, PREPARED WITH TAP WATER	0	0	0	0	6 FL OZ
30	BREAKFAST	CREAM, HEAVY	104	0	12	0	2 TBSP.
30	*BREAKFAST*	*TOTAL*	*1,458*	*52*	*121*	*23*	
30	LUNCH	**OMELET**					
30	LUNCH	▷ 2 MEDIUM EGG, WHOLE, COOKED, OMELET	160	11	7	0	1 SERVING
30	LUNCH	▷ CHEESE, CHEDDAR	220	14	18	4	2 OZ

DAILY SMART MEAL PLANS

Day	Meal	Food Description	Calories	Proteins	Fat	Net Carbs	Serving Size
30	LUNCH	▷ AVOCADOS, RAW, CALIFORNIA	192	3	18	2	1/2 CUP
30	LUNCH	BREAD, LOW CARB	60	6	2	1	1 SLICE, 1 OZ
30	LUNCH	BUTTER, SALTED	102	0	12	0	1 TBSP.
30	LUNCH	WATER	0	0	0	0	8 FL OZ
30	*LUNCH*	*TOTAL*	*734*	*34*	*57*	*7*	
30	DINNER	**TUNA SALAD**					
30	DINNER	▷ TUNA, WHITE, CANNED IN OIL SOLIDS	316	46	14	0	6 OZ
30	DINNER	▷ MAYONNAISE DRESSING	206	0	24	0	2 TBSP.
30	DINNER	▷ PICKLE RELISH, SWEET	20	0	0	5	1 TBSP.
30	DINNER	▷ ONIONS, COOKED	7	0	0	2	1 TBSP.
30	DINNER	▷ CELERY, RAW	8	1	0	1	1/2 CUP
30	DINNER	MELONS, CASABA, RAW	48	2	0	9	1 CUP
30	DINNER	TEA, BLACK, BREWED, ICED	2	0	0	1	8 FL OZ
30	*DINNER*	*TOTAL*	*607*	*49*	*38*	*18*	
31	BREAKFAST	**TAHINI WRAP**					
31	BREAKFAST	▷ SESAME BUTTER, TAHINI, FROM ROASTED AND TOASTED KERNELS (MOST COMMON TYPE)	178	6	16	4	2 TBSP.
31	BREAKFAST	▷ CHEESE, PARMESAN, HARD	220	20	14	2	2 OZ
31	BREAKFAST	▷ TORTILLAS, LOW CARB, WHOLE WHEAT, FLOUR	90	3	2	3	1 TORTILLA, 28G
31	BREAKFAST	HIBISCUS TEA	0	0	0	0	8 FL OZ
31	*BREAKFAST*	*TOTAL*	*488*	*29*	*32*	*9*	

DAILY SMART MEAL PLANS

Day	Meal	Food Description	Calories	Proteins	Fat	Net Carbs	Serving Size
31	LUNCH	**CHICKEN WRAP**					
31	LUNCH	▷ CHICKEN, BROILER, ROTISSERIE, GRILLED, BREAST MEAT AND SKIN	149	22	7	0	3 OZ
31	LUNCH	▷ CHEESE, CREAM	96	2	10	2	2 TBSP.
31	LUNCH	▷ LETTUCE, BUTTERHEAD (INCLUDES BOSTON AND BIBB TYPES), RAW	7	1	0	0	1 CUP
31	LUNCH	MACADAMIA NUTS, DRY ROASTED	474	5	50	4	1/2 CUP
31	LUNCH	HIBISCUS TEA	0	0	0	0	8 FL OZ
31	*LUNCH*	*TOTAL*	*726*	*30*	*67*	*6*	
31	DINNER	VEGETARIAN FILLETS	494	40	30	6	2 FILLET
31	DINNER	CHEESE, GOAT, SEMISOFT TYPE	408	24	32	0	4 OZ
31	DINNER	ASPARAGUS, COOKED	32	5	1	0	1 CUP
31	DINNER	COFFEE, BREWED FROM GROUNDS, PREPARED WITH TAP WATER	0	0	0	0	6 FL OZ
31	DINNER	CREAM, HEAVY	104	0	12	0	2 TBSP.
31	*DINNER*	*TOTAL*	*1,038*	*69*	*75*	*6*	
32	BREAKFAST	YOGURT, PLAIN, WHOLE MILK	170	10	8	14	1 CUP
32	BREAKFAST	CHEESE, GRUYERE	232	16	18	0	2 OZ
32	BREAKFAST	WATER	0	0	0	0	8 FL OZ
32	*BREAKFAST*	*TOTAL*	*402*	*26*	*26*	*14*	
32	LUNCH	**STEAK WITH ONIONS AND MUSHROOMS**					
32	LUNCH	▷ BEEF, LOIN, TOP LOIN STEAK	448	44	30	0	6 OZ
32	LUNCH	▷ ONIONS, YELLOW, SAUTÉED	115	1	9	6	1 CUP
32	LUNCH	▷ MUSHROOMS, WHITE, RAW	21	3	0	2	1 CUP
32	LUNCH	▷ BUTTER, SALTED	204	0	24	0	2 TBSP.

DAILY SMART MEAL PLANS

Day	Meal	Food Description	Calories	Proteins	Fat	Net Carbs	Serving Size
32	LUNCH	TEA, BLACK, BREWED, ICED	2	0	0	1	8 FL OZ
32	*LUNCH*	*TOTAL*	*790*	*48*	*63*	*9*	
32	DINNER	**GRILLED PORTABELLA**					
32	DINNER	▷ MUSHROOMS, PORTABELLA, GRILLED	70	8	2	4	2 CUP
32	DINNER	▷ CHEESE, MOZZARELLA, WHOLE MILK	340	24	24	4	4 OZ
32	DINNER	**SALAD**					
32	DINNER	▷ LETTUCE, RED LEAF, RAW	4	0	0	1	1 CUP
32	DINNER	▷ AVOCADOS, RAW, CALIFORNIA	384	5	35	4	1 CUP
32	DINNER	▷ CHEESE, MONTEREY	211	14	17	1	4 OZ
32	DINNER	▷ SALAD DRESSING, RANCH DRESSING	63	0	7	1	1 TBSP.
32	DINNER	TEA, BLACK, BREWED, ICED	2	0	0	1	8 FL OZ
32	*DINNER*	*TOTAL*	*1,074*	*51*	*85*	*16*	
33	BREAKFAST	**CHEESE WRAP**					
33	BREAKFAST	▷ CHEESE, COTTAGE, CREAMED, LARGE OR SMALL CURD	111	13	5	4	4 OZ
33	BREAKFAST	▷ CHEESE, PASTEURIZED PROCESS, CHEDDAR OR AMERICAN, LOW SODIUM	213	13	18	1	1/2 CUP, CUBED
33	BREAKFAST	▷ TORTILLAS, LOW CARB, WHOLE WHEAT, FLOUR	90	3	2	3	1 TORTILLA, 28G
33	BREAKFAST	WATER	0	0	0	0	8 FL OZ
33	*BREAKFAST*	*TOTAL*	*414*	*29*	*25*	*8*	
33	LUNCH	**CHILI**					
33	LUNCH	▷ CHILI NO BEANS, CANNED SOUP	200	10	15	6	1/2 CUP
33	LUNCH	▷ CHEESE, MEXICAN, QUESO QUESADILLA	400	28	32	0	4 OZ
33	LUNCH	WATER	0	0	0	0	8 FL OZ

DAILY SMART MEAL PLANS

Day	Meal	Food Description	Calories	Proteins	Fat	Net Carbs	Serving Size
33	*LUNCH*	*TOTAL*	*600*	*38*	*47*	*6*	
33	DINNER	**ALMOND BUTTER SANDWICH**					
33	DINNER	▷ ALMOND BUTTER, PLAIN	392	12	36	4	4 TBSP.
33	DINNER	▷ BREAD, LOW CARB	120	12	4	2	2 SLICE, 1 OZ
33	DINNER	SPINACH, COOKED, BOILED	41	5	0	3	1 CUP
33	DINNER	CHEESE, SWISS	502	36	37	7	1 CUP, CUBED
33	DINNER	SPARKLING WATER	0	0	0	0	8 FL OZ
33	*DINNER*	*TOTAL*	*1,055*	*65*	*77*	*16*	
34	BREAKFAST	ALMOND BUTTER, PLAIN	196	6	18	2	2 TBSP.
34	BREAKFAST	CRACKERS, LOW CARB	100	4	7	6	10 CRACKERS
34	BREAKFAST	EGG, WHOLE, COOKED, HARD-BOILED	211	17	14	2	1 CUP
34	BREAKFAST	WATER	0	0	0	0	8 FL OZ
34	*BREAKFAST*	*TOTAL*	*507*	*27*	*39*	*10*	
34	LUNCH	PORK, LOIN, TENDERLOIN	171	25	7	0	3 OZ
34	LUNCH	**SALAD**					
34	LUNCH	▷ LETTUCE, BUTTERHEAD (INCLUDES BOSTON AND BIBB TYPES), RAW	7	1	0	0	1 CUP
34	LUNCH	▷ SPINACH, RAW	7	1	0	0	1 CUP
34	LUNCH	▷ ONIONS, SPRING OR SCALLIONS (INCLUDES TOPS AND BULB), RAW	16	1	0	2	1/2 CUP
34	LUNCH	▷ TOMATOES, RED CHERRY, RAW	14	1	0	2	1/2 CUP
34	LUNCH	▷ PECANS, DRY ROASTED	199	3	21	1	1 OZ

DAILY SMART MEAL PLANS

Day	Meal	Food Description	Calories	Proteins	Fat	Net Carbs	Serving Size
34	LUNCH	▷ SALAD DRESSING, THOUSAND ISLAND	122	0	12	4	2 TBSP.
34	LUNCH	WATER	0	0	0	0	8 FL OZ
34	LUNCH	TOTAL	536	32	40	9	
34	DINNER	SAUSAGE, CHICKEN AND BEEF, SMOKED	407	26	33	0	1 CUP
34	DINNER	**SALAD**					
34	DINNER	▷ LETTUCE, RED LEAF, RAW	4	0	0	1	1 CUP
34	DINNER	▷ AVOCADOS, RAW, CALIFORNIA	384	5	35	4	1 CUP
34	DINNER	▷ CHEESE, MOZZARELLA, WHOLE MILK	170	12	12	2	2 OZ
34	DINNER	▷ MUSHROOMS, WHITE, RAW	21	3	0	2	1 CUP
34	DINNER	▷ SALAD DRESSING, SESAME SEED DRESSING	132	0	14	2	2 TBSP.
34	DINNER	WINE, TABLE, RED, MERLOT	122	0	0	4	5 FL OZ
34	DINNER	TOTAL	1,240	46	94	15	
35	BREAKFAST	**CHICKEN WRAP**					
35	BREAKFAST	▷ CHICKEN BREAST, DELI, ROTISSERIE SEASONED, SLICED, PREPACKAGED	48	8	0	0	4 SLICES
35	BREAKFAST	▷ LETTUCE, BUTTERHEAD (INCLUDES BOSTON AND BIBB TYPES), RAW	7	1	0	0	1 CUP
35	BREAKFAST	▷ CHEESE, GOAT, SEMISOFT TYPE	408	24	32	0	4 OZ
35	BREAKFAST	▷ SALAD DRESSING, RANCH DRESSING	63	0	7	1	1 TBSP.
35	BREAKFAST	COFFEE, BREWED FROM GROUNDS, PREPARED WITH TAP WATER	0	0	0	0	6 FL OZ
35	BREAKFAST	CREAM, HEAVY	104	0	12	0	2 TBSP.
35	BREAKFAST	TOTAL	630	33	51	1	

DAILY SMART MEAL PLANS

Day	Meal	Food Description	Calories	Proteins	Fat	Net Carbs	Serving Size
35	LUNCH	**GRILLED CHEESE**					
35	LUNCH	▷ CHEESE, CHEDDAR	440	28	36	8	4 OZ
35	LUNCH	▷ BREAD, LOW CARB	120	12	4	2	2 SLICE, 1 OZ
35	LUNCH	▷ BUTTER, SALTED	204	0	24	0	2 TBSP.
35	LUNCH	COFFEE, BREWED FROM GROUNDS, PREPARED WITH TAP WATER	0	0	0	0	6 FL OZ
35	LUNCH	CREAM, HEAVY	104	0	12	0	2 TBSP.
35	*LUNCH*	*TOTAL*	*868*	*40*	*76*	*10*	
35	DINNER	TURKEY, BREAST, MEAT AND SKIN, ROASTED	278	50	10	0	6 OZ
35	DINNER	TURKEY GRAVY, CANNED, READY-TO-SERVE	16	0	0	2	2 TBSP.
35	DINNER	BRUSSELS SPROUTS, COOKED	65	6	1	7	1 CUP
35	DINNER	ALFREDO CREAM SAUCE	228	6	26	2	2 OZ
35	DINNER	TEA, BLACK, BREWED	2	0	0	1	6 FL OZ
35	DINNER	CREAM, HEAVY	104	0	12	0	2 TBSP.
35	*DINNER*	*TOTAL*	*693*	*62*	*49*	*12*	

Low-Carb Tortilla Snacks

I think when I discovered low-carb tortillas I felt just like Columbus when he landed in the New World (lucky and happy). I found a bread substitute that is Nirvana on a low, controlled-carb eating plan. I try to eat very few wheat products, but I do concede to a few low-carb tortillas. I use them for sandwiches and wraps—and even broil them to make chips for dipping! Here are some of my favorite fillings for these tasty tortillas:

- Cold cuts
- Cheese
- Salsa
- Low-carb cheese spreads
- Chicken salad
- Turkey salad
- Tuna salad
- Shrimp, crab, or lobster salads
- Egg salad
- Melted ham and cheese
- Hot dogs, brats, and hamburgers
- Sour cream (with berries, stevia and also as famous onion dip with soup mix)

Five Weeks of SMaRT Eating Tips

Any time you start a new health or diet plan, it can be hard to adjust. Often as you change your eating habits, you encounter different challenges during different phases of your program. I've compiled some helpful tips below, specific to each of the five weeks in the metabolic makeover plan.

Week One

As you begin your first week on the program, hopefully the menu ideas above will help get you started and make it easier but they are suggestions only. The most important aspect of these meal plans is that carbohydrates are the foods with the least wiggle room. Independent of size and activity level, carbohydrates *must* be controlled on The SMaRT Diet. The specific portions are based on a person who is minimally active, slightly overweight, and about 160 pounds. Many involved in the Metabolic Makeover Program are larger and more active, and their respective calorie count will probably be higher than the numbers presented in these daily menus.

Remember, you can *always* substitute "like" foods, including eating more fats and proteins (therefore more calories or fewer if you don't feel like eating that much) if you have that inclination but not carbs! So pick your carbohydrate level (20 grams daily for a strict ketogenic limitation or 40 grams daily to start the carb controlled program) and work around that with your fats and proteins.

If you like or prefer certain foods that are low in carbohydrates, don't be shy. Eat them all you want! I sometimes eat steak and bunless hamburgers as my main food source for days at a time. Sometimes I get on an egg jag and eat egg dishes for breakfast and dinner for many days in a row. As long as the guidelines are met for each food category (carbs, fats, proteins), you have all the latitude you want for amounts and selections of foods as well as meals per day. It helps to eat the foods you like, because it will make it easier to stick to the program. So if you don't like fish, don't force yourself to eat it. Eat chicken instead. Or if you hate kale, eat spinach, arugula, or mixed greens. The best part about The SMaRT Diet is that there is a lot of flexibility, so eat what you enjoy!

You may encounter some common hurdles at the beginning of the program. Some people feel a strong urge to have bread or pasta. It's a normal "carb withdrawal." It should be noted that carbohydrates trigger opiate responses in the brain. In short, they can be chemically addictive. I have found that women seem to be more inclined or disposed to this condition. There is also a condition termed "Atkins flu." It is described by some as a vague feeling of lack of energy and not being "right"—slight nausea, headache, and so on. This circumstance is usually associated with sugar fluctuations and actual carbohydrate withdrawal, which translates into your body telling you it is used to sugar and it no longer has this fuel source to rely upon. The bright side is that your body is also telling you that it is about to transition into fat burning. So it's worth toughing out a little in most cases.

Week Two

By now, you should be starting to get the feel of the SMaRT eating plan. You may already have it down to your liking or you may still be trying to find your eating niche. Try to figure out what works or what gives you a problem. Some folks are very carbohydrate sensitive. Even a small amount of "acceptable" levels of carbohydrate consumption can trigger *the drive for more (carbs)*. My suggestion is to try to eat your favorite things that fit into the plan. You can even go forward (at any time during the plan) and look at future week's meal plans to see if one or two particularly catch your eye.

If you're doing well, stick with it. If you're having some problems or feel uncertain about the eating plan, do some real planning and make it your "job" to get it right. The more prepared you are, the more likely you will stick with it and succeed. Be sure to keep healthy, low-carb food options in your house. And, if possible, eliminate the temptations. It's worth it, and it does take some more time with some people than others. You ARE on the SMaRT path to losing fat and changing your metabolism for good!

Week Three

By now almost everyone engaged in the SMaRT plan can see and measure significant differences in pants size and feel, energy levels, the appearance of some muscle shape, and a good feeling of satisfying eating. Hopefully, you are impressed with the power of two fifteen-minute workouts and eating without fretting over counting calories. Hopefully, this will encourage you to stick with it.

You should have developed a pattern of eating that suits you and fits into your schedule and lifestyle. Some folks have little slips off the wagon, but that's human nature. The way you handle these will go a long way in determining long-term success and metabolic turnaround. Don't let one bad meal choice ruin an entire day—or week for that matter. If this process was so easy, everyone would do it and I wouldn't have written this book. KEEP PLUGGIN!

Week Four

At this point in time, you should have a good idea of how to shop, cook, and organize your food selections. You might have favorites for meals and snacks ready to go when you need or want them. Hopefully, you will be less inclined to have cravings triggered by special events, commercials on TV, or while shopping.

At this point, it is not uncommon to be able to fiddle with carb counting. Some folks can gradually and subtly increase carb intake if they want to. Some much prefer their sense of health and well-being in their strict low-carb state and remain on that track. It is not uncommon for people who only need to lose 5 to 10 pounds to be close to their goal and want to experiment with slight carb increases (maybe more berries, nuts, dark chocolate, or similar treats while still keeping track of their carb content). Many people get into checking ketones with urine strips and blood sugar with a glucometer. These are great, objective methods for keeping track of the chemical effects that your behaviors are having on your metabolism. You should have some metabolic "momentum" garnered at this point, so enjoy the ride and stay determined! Only one more week!

Week Five

You are now in the homestretch. At this point in the process, you will have likely fallen off the wagon for a day or two. Additionally, you will have developed your own diet preferences and patterns, discovering what agrees with your lifestyle and palatable behaviors. If you've been pretty steady in your application of the SMaRT nutritional component as well as the twice a week exercise regimen, it might be a good time to have some lab work or other measurements done. You will probably see significant, measurable changes in your body.

I suggest writing down some major elements you have learned to be most successful in your program and try to reinforce those habits by planning ahead to keep them going. I have found that many of the long-term success stories revolve around repeated, consistent applications of eating the same way and scheduling exercise and activities in the same weekly patterns. These are the foundations for long-term metabolic change and feeling and looking better than you would have believed five weeks ago. Great Job!

While the five-week metabolic makeover plan is a set timeline to get you started on a 10-pound fat loss, there's no reason not to keep going. By now you have likely changed many of your eating habits, and it will be easier to continue a healthy SMaRT diet and exercise plan

Dr. Ben's Lifetime Meal Tips

- Shop for and keep handy "go to" foods to eat. I keep pepperoni, cold cuts, nuts, eggs, cheese, and roasted chicken on board at all times.

- Plan your meals a day or two ahead: meats thawed, veggies on hand, and even perhaps packaged for lunch or travel for the next few days.

- If you know you're going out to eat, try to figure out your menu. Don't be shy to tell prospective hosts that you're eating low carb and that means meat, fish, poultry, and veggies. They should be able to accommodate those guidelines.

- I found some precooked hamburgers that can be microwaved in 2–3 minutes. Believe it or not, they're pretty good. It's helpful to find easy meals like this for days when you are too busy to cook.

- Low-carb tortillas save the day when it comes to low-carb bread substitutes. I wrap all kinds of meats and salads (tuna, chicken, egg, shrimp) into these. I even make my Italian sausage with sautéed onions and peppers and put them into these low-carb delights.

- Sour cream is another great, high-fat, low-carb food. You can make onion or veggie dip for low carb-tortillas (broiled to make chips) and chopped vegetables. You can also use some Splenda or other sugar substitute in sour cream for a dessert. With a little bit of carb allowance, you can have berries and cream, using sour cream.

- Low-carb Jello is another great treat with some real whipped cream.

- Discover some treats and crunchy things that fit into your carb scheme, enjoy yourself, and eat well until satisfied and smiley! Stay Healthy.

Monitoring Blood Sugar Levels

Since one of our major concerns and efforts is the regulation and control of our blood sugar levels and responses, it has proven helpful for many to purchase a glucometer. Glucometers are simple devices that measure blood sugar (glucose) levels. They can be purchased at any pharmacy without a prescription and usually cost between $15 and $30. They require test strips, which can be costly but can be purchased more economically online. I would suggest shopping around for test strips a little to get the best deal. I use a "Nova Max Plus" glucometer and test strips.

This process requires a simple finger prick (pen usually provided in package). The two most representative readings can be taken upon waking; these are called fasting glucose. Most literature indicates that a reading less than 100 is fine. The next (second) critical reading should be taken one hour after first starting a meal, not two hours and not after the meal is completed. This is the time at which the initial insulin response to a meal can be most sensitively calculated. That number is commonly agreed to be below 140 if carbohydrates are ingested or 120 if you are sticking to a controlled-carb plan. Please remember that these are *general* norms. Each of us might respond out of the suggested range. However, if you do, I would suggest that you ask your doctor to order a Hemoglobin A-1C blood test. This measurement represents the three-month average of glucose in your blood protein (hemoglobin) that turns over on the average in about 90 days. This is a strong representation of the status of the glucose/ insulin axis of metabolism.

Ketostix Test Strips

Among other useful tools for keeping track of your metabolic responses to controlled-carb eating are ketostix test strips. Many familiar with the Atkins diet remember that these strips are used to measure ketones in the urine. Ketones are molecules that result from the breakdown of fat. When more fat is being used as fuel than normal (usually a good thing for folks interested in reducing fat), ketone levels will rise, and they can be measured by these simple test strips available in any drug store. Since the body produces two major types of ketones—beta-hydroxybutyrate and acetoacetate—the results do not tell the whole story but in most cases can be useful motivational tools to keep low-carb eaters on track.

Should I Take Vitamins and Minerals?

It is reasonable to ask about vitamin and mineral supplementation. We have been so inundated with the business and propaganda of the supplement business and the "health" food industry that we have very little rational understanding of supplementation. My first point of advice is to worry less about this issue than we are led to believe. Very few Americans suffer bona fide vitamin deficiencies. However, since most of our food sources are less nutritionally dense than they had been at a previous time in our history, simple vitamin and mineral supplementation is probably prudent. Again, in my experience and opinion, it really can't hurt in the overwhelming majority of cases.

You can make yourself absolutely bleary-eyed trying to read and distinguish the claims of vitamin and mineral ingestion. Don't forget there are academic folks who've spent most of their professional lives studying some micro-nutrient (a vitamin or mineral). So here's my take, determined by substantial review and practical clinical experience: The Eades, authors of *Protein Power*, whom I respect greatly, suggest 1 gram of vitamin C, vitamin D(3) 50 IU (the 2013 RDA is stated as 600 IU per day), Beta carotene (vitamin A) 25 IU, and B complex, including folic acid and vitamin E (D-alpha tocopherol). They also recommend mineral supplementation. This combination can be found in KAL-High Potency Soft Multiple Vitamin, Twinlab-Dual Tab Sustained Release Mega Vitamin and

Mineral Formula, or Mega Food Vitamin and Mineral. If these are not readily available, simply talk to the seller to see if they can provide reasonable comparisons.

Dr. Ben's Favorite Low-Carb Meals

I am what people refer to as a "very good" eater. Translation: I have a large capacity for food volume. Always have. I LOVE to eat. One of the motivations for me studying the art and science of eating is driven by my predilection for EATING! When I was younger, I would go to "all you can eat" buffets and have been asked to leave without paying in more than one location. I recently went to my favorite steak joint with my friend Charles Barkley (yes, that Charles Barkley), and he said, "B (his nickname for me), how BIG is your stomach?" I laughed and said, "You ain't doin' too bad yourself, 4X" (that was his shirt size at the time). I still consume large quantities of low-carb foods. Following are some of my favorite ideas and recipes for good, controlled-carb snacks and meals.

I LOVE pepperoni! I keep it everywhere (my first aid kit). I eat it whenever I feel the munchies or want to add some real zesty flavor to a meal. There are all sorts of salamis that may also fit into this description for you.

Nuts are another favorite, but you have to be mindful because they're so easy to gobble in huge volumes, and they can carry a higher than desired carb load at that level. My Famous Nut Mix (the BEST) includes: Mixed, deluxe, salted nuts, salted cashews, salted macadamias, and seasoned almonds. My favorite seasoned almonds are the soy/wasabi and jalapeño. I usually put them in a big gallon Ziploc bag (don't forget to ZIP it!) and then I roll them around until they form a good mix. You won't believe how good these are! I really should patent these!

Since I'm Italian, I love my Italian dishes. One of my favorites is sausage, peppers, and onions wrapped in my low-carb tortillas (you can even eat this without the tortilla). I like spicy Italian sausage, but you can use sweet or mild if you don't like spicy foods. I usually cook them on the grill. I cut up the onions and bell peppers in slices—I try to use an assortment of colors. I sauté the veggies with garlic in a pan of olive oil until they are more cooked than stir-fried crunchy, but you can cook them to your preference. Add a little salt and some Tabasco sauce to really jazz it up.

Dr. Ben's "Granma's Chicken": Cut up a whole chicken into small pieces or simply get the best parts for you. I use thighs because they're easy and have lots of flavor and fat. Brown the chicken in a pan with garlic and olive oil. Season with salt, oregano, and onion powder. Place browned chicken pieces in a crock pot and coat with tomato paste and add wine (optional), and let it stew on low for a few hours (literally 3 or 4 to overnight). This is a spectacular, tasty dish. I usually have salad or veggies with it to make a nice Italian feast!

When I'm craving "breaded" chicken, veal, or pork cutlets, I make a low-carb version. I take any boneless cut of meat and pound it flat. Then I dip them in some egg and roll them in Parmesan cheese and either a very small amount of breadcrumb (check carb count) or diced walnuts for a low-carb form of breadcrumb. I add some oregano, onion powder, and salt. I fry them in olive oil with fresh chopped garlic. When you get to a level of slightly increasing carbs, you can add some tomato sauce and grated mozzarella cheese to these cutlets and, viola, chicken parm!

I grill meats of all kinds, but I marinate the meat for a day or two. For my marinade I use olive oil, balsamic vinegar (check carbs) or seasoned rice wine vinegar, oregano, salt, garlic, and onion powder. I put everything together in a Ziploc bag and place it in the fridge for a couple of days, rotating the meat once in awhile. Never overcook your meats. Once you take them off grill, they continue to cook a little. Don't forget.

I also love to sauté my vegetables in garlic and olive oil and add grated Parmesan cheese to the mix. Sometimes I add a small amount of breadcrumb or diced walnuts. Makes veggies a real treat!

I love garden salads, because you can put just about anything in them (as long as it's low carb). In addition to various forms of greens and lettuce, I love artichoke hearts, cherry tomatoes, bacon bits, sunflower seeds, sliced almonds, Parmesan cheese, shredded cheddar or mozzarella, and pepperoni slices. You can also make a good Cobb salad by adding slices of cheese, meats, and egg. This can be a real delicious meal in itself. I make my own salad dressing, using olive oil, any kind of vinegar (check carbs), garlic powder, onion powder, oregano, salt (optional: black pepper, crushed red pepper), and I always sprinkle my Parmesan cheese liberally.

• • •

Many of the "ideas" about eating that were taught to us by well-meaning parents, grandparents, teachers, and other supposedly reliable sources were simply folklore and myth. Don't worry about abiding by the nutritional "rules" we all held so dearly: eating three "square" meals a day, varying the foods that we eat, eating a "good" breakfast, and so on. I'm so skeptical that I'm not even sure if the one about not going in the water until an hour after lunch holds much of the aforementioned water. In any case, my experience tells me that you are best served by developing your own plan or niche when it comes to what works best regarding your eating selection and pattern.

The most relevant factor in food selection is how you respond as demonstrated by energy levels and desired body composition. Do you feel hungry often? Are you gaining or losing weight (fat) when you don't want to? These are your keys for dietary assessment. Based on years of scientific research and hands-on practice, I know that you will have positive results in both fat loss and increased energy if you follow my controlled-carbohydrate plan. Now that we've covered the essentials of the metabolic makeover both in exercise and diet, we'll cover some specific topics of interest in Part III of the book.

Topics of Interest for Participants in Weight Loss and Exercise Programs

CHAPTER EIGHT

MEN, WOMEN, AND WEIGHT LOSS

When it comes to the topic of weight loss, I'm often asked about the "difference" between men and women—almost always by women. It seems unfair to many wives that their husbands can lose weight more easily than they can themselves. You frequently hear stories of women who've been dieting and exercising for months, only to lose a few pounds while their significant other starts a similar program and loses 10 pounds within a month. When I first began working in this field during the early 1970s, the domain of exercise was absolutely male territory. I designed programs for fairly elite athletes, macho men, and hard-core workout guys. I honestly didn't think about women wanting to do high intensity training. That's really the way it was! Shortly after I started my practice, a couple of gals came in to begin to train. One was a model and the other was a world-class volleyball player. I explained that I was going to treat and train them just like everyone else. They agreed. That's when I learned that women could kick butt just like the guys.

Since that time, I have handled many cases and read and studied hundreds of thousands of pages of research, mostly in academic settings. Some of the material is relevant and helpful, but much of it is just plain silly and possibly insulting. In any case, for the most part, men and women behave similarly with regard to exercise and eating, but I must admit that women can be a little more metabolically complex.

Common Weight Challenges for Women

Not all tendencies in the realm of health and wellness are easily and definitively explained. Here are a few assumptions and observations regarding the complexity of female weight gain/loss issues:

- Approximately 1 in 10 women of childbearing age have polycystic ovary syndrome (PCOS). In addition to causing ovulation problems and infertility, PCOS can cause insulin resistance, often associated with excess fat storage, especially around the waist.

- Women suffer a higher incidence of depression than men and related conditions (to depression) have been shown to produce an excess of stress hormones (including cortisol) that are connected to increased retention of abdominal fat.

- Progesterone is another female hormone that can drive weight gain and conversely inhibit weight loss when its proportions to other hormones become imbalanced or out of ideal ratios with other sex hormones.

- Women also tend to suffer from higher incidences of allergies and gastro-intestinal problems, including gluten intolerance and leaky gut syndrome, which are sometimes difficult to diagnose but certainly connected to problematic weight-gain issues.

- The consequences of some birth control prescriptions are also associated with common weight control symptoms in a fair percentage of the women who take them.

- Women are 5 to 8 times more likely to manifest thyroid problems than men (American Thyroid Association). One of the major roles of the thyroid gland is the control of energy use and storage. This hormone's role is vital in the quest for weight loss.

Any of the above situations can dramatically affect weight loss and health, thus making it harder for women to lose weight and keep it off.

Non-Gender Characteristics

Much of the differential between the male and female responses to diet and exercise can be explained by some non-gender characteristics, such as body size, lean body mass, and corresponding metabolic rate. In simple terms, one would assume logically that a 200-pound person would lose more weight, more quickly, than a 120-pound person. That describes some of the difference between men and women, since men are generally larger. Secondarily, but just as significant, men usually have more lean mass than most women, much of which is muscle tissue. That's significant because it means that men need more energy to support the metabolic demand of this extra muscle and that they have more sites for insulin reception or use. Skeletal muscle houses a large number of our insulin receptors, and having more of them reduces the likelihood of insulin resistance, which leads to a myriad of weight-related problems.

Even though these body size and muscle discrepancies can explain some of the differences between the genders, it does *not* explain the observed totality of the dichotomy of exercise and diet responses. In my experience, it appears that there is some hormonal complexity affecting female metabolism that does not occur with their male counterparts.

Women's Weight Issues

My own research and experience, as well as the research of some women's health specialists in the field, points to a number of women-specific weight issues. They include hormonal imbalances, neurotransmitter imbalances, digestive imbalances, systemic inflammation, and liver taxation. We'll take a look at why and how these imbalances occur and how to counteract them.

Thyroid Imbalance

One of the most common hormonal issues in women is related to the thyroid, which can have a strong impact on the ability to successfully lose weight. Dr. Fox, a woman's health expert, explains: "If TSH (Thyroid Stimulating Hormone) increased over time, weight was more likely to go up." In a study that Dr. Fox was involved in, they divided the patients into four groups, from those whose TSH increased the least to those whose TSH increased the most. Women whose TSH changed the most gained 2.3 kilograms (about 5 pounds on average). Some gained more. Dr. Fox found a similar pattern in men, although the increases were less significant. The men whose TSH increased the most gained on average 1.3 kilograms or nearly 3 pounds over the three-and-a-half-year follow-up. The study was a two-year follow-up of data from the Framingham research of 2,400 participants who had normal thyroid readings but indicated that the movement or trajectory of TSH levels correlated to weight gain over the long term. The simple take-away from this information is that thyroid function should be followed not only by simple T3 and T4 indices but also by following the trajectory of TSH.

The study, along with two other recent reports about the association, provides interesting information, according to Roy E. Weiss, MD, PhD, the Rabbi Morris Esformes Professor of Adult and Pediatric Endocrinology, Diabetes, and Metabolism at the University of Chicago Medical Center. He coauthored an editorial to accompany the study. "What may be within the normal range [of thyroid functioning] for a population may not be the normal thyroid levels for a particular individual," he tells WebMD. The exact mechanisms for this weight gain are not clearly established at this time but provide another potential indicator to be followed by those concerned with "hard to lose" weight gain. In my experience, this is a very important concept: "Normal" is population-oriented information, which can differ greatly on an individual basis. I often suggest that folks get a baseline set of lab work done as early in life as possible (in their 20s or 30s). That information will lend much more credibility to subsequent lab test information gathered later in life. In simple terms, "relative" high or low lab numbers might very well be healthy and normal for you as an individual. Changes in lab numbers, on the other hand, might be much more significant than the absolute numbers based on population "norms."

Ramachandran S. Vasan, MD, another coauthor of a thyroid study and a professor of medicine at Boston University, notes: "While we show an association, we can't claim cause and effect." While it may be tempting to blame the thyroid when weight increases, weight gain has many causes, according to Dr. Fox.

Adrenal Problems Related to Weight Gain/Weight-loss Resistance

There is no question that the compromised function of the adrenal glands can cause many problems associated with weight gain and stubborn resistance to its loss. In fact, some of the following symptoms are frequently caused by adrenal "insufficiency"—but not always Robert Vigersky, MD, a past president of the Endocrine Society, says the symptoms of adrenal problems are very common in people in general. Though people often blame their hormonal glands, such as the adrenals or thyroid, for their tiredness, Vigersky says in many cases fatigue is due to other common problems. All of the following can affect your energy level without involving your adrenal glands.

- **Poor sleep habits.** A large body of research concludes that sleep is a vital element in a healthy lifestyle. Poor sleep has been associated with exaggerated insulin resistance, weight gain, increased cortisol secretion, and a host of associated health problems. Coincidentally, the reduced levels of inflammation associated with low-carb eating and properly applied high intensity exercise (SMaRT) greatly support "good" restorative sleeping patterns. Also, high intensity exercise promotes the secretion of IGF-1, a growth promoting signaling protein that is strongly associated with healthy sleep levels called "REM" sleep.

- **Poor diet.** It has been presented significantly in this book that low-carb eating comprises a most healthy nutritional approach. Enough said!

- **Stress at work or home.** In my experience, stress is a most elusive and pervasive element of human behavior to define. In any case, it has appeared to me that "physical" stress is appropriately addressed and handled well by "controlled exercise stress." The response to SMaRT training is real muscular fatigue and metabolic (chemical) stimulation, driving an upsurge response in muscular energy and work capacity. That's a "good," healthy cycle of stress and response. The brain response to high intensity exercise promotes up-regulation (increases) in two chemicals called "neurotransmitters." They are norepinephrine and dopamine. Norepinephrine makes signals to the brain "stronger," and dopamine makes signals to the brain "clearer" (reduces the "static"). As a practical explanation, kids with ADHD or folks with Alzheimer's disease and Parkinson's all demonstrate lowered levels of these two vital chemicals. These neurotransmitters are simultaneously associated with anxiety issues, which logically lead to "stressful" situations and conditions.

- **Depression.** According to Dr. John Ratey, author of *Spark,* almost 20 million people suffer from diagnosed depression in the US. Most of them are women. In Great Britain, exercise is being used as a frontline treatment mechanism for depression. Once again, higher intensity exercise produces higher levels of "good brain chemistry" than lower, but even at a steady state, lower level of exercise or activity, depression levels can be significantly reduced.

Neurotransmitter Imbalance

As stated in the previous section, a neurotransmitter imbalance can be strongly and effectively addressed by the application of real exercise (SMaRT). In sophisticated brain imaging, the "growth" of areas of the brain that regulate mood, cognitive skills, and anxiety actually occurs as a result of structured exercise. Again the levels of norepinephrine and dopamine (prominent neurotransmitters) are significantly enhanced by exercise. I strongly advise interested parties, including physicians and therapists, to read *Spark* by John Ratey. It is a wonderfully informative work, and I plan to advise Dr. Ratey about some of the subtleties of exercise and superior benefits of high intensity programs.

Digestive Imbalance

The bibles regarding digestion, eating, and weight gain/loss in my readings have been *Wheat Belly* by Dr. William Davis and *Grain Brain* by Dr. David Perlmutter. Davis contends that since the inception of the "new" wheat strains around the 1950s, human consumption has increased, and the genetic constitution of the newer hybridized grain was not something humans were even vaguely genetically geared to handle. He suggests that since bread/wheat products are the most highly consumed in conventional, modern diets, the elimination of these will go a long way in alleviating associated nutritional ailments, including obesity and diabetes. Perlmutter, in *Grain Brain* and *Brain Maker,* contends that the proteins as well as the carbohydrates in grains act as inhibitors of normal brain health and cell turnover.

In *Brain Maker,* Perlmutter contends that the biome (the state of the gut bacteria) has everything to do with regulating metabolism, including fat storage and usage. Carbohydrate foods have a tendency to ferment (that's why one makes alcohol out of fruits and not meat). That fermentation can instigate all sorts of upheaval in the normal, healthy state of the flora of the human gut. The ensuing repercussions can certainly lead to weight problems and other metabolic disorders. Again, for unknown reasons, women are much more likely to suffer from leaky gut and other gastro-intestinal disorders than men. The reasons are proposed to emanate from social and behavioral differences (internalizing stresses), rather than physiological differences in men and women.

Systemic Inflammation

The topic of inflammation has been broached before in chapter one when discussing our body's chemistry during exercise. However, the common state of inflammation is so prominent in association with weight-related conditions that it should be reinforced. It was generally accepted that being overweight or obese caused inflammatory responses that led to diabetes, heart disease, stroke, arthritis, some forms of cancer, and so on. It is now generally accepted that the state of inflammation triggers these degenerative disorders. We had it backwards and, as a result, many of the protocols were wild swings in the dark. They didn't work. We have more ammunition now, and we should be better at addressing these pervasive problems.

Another note on differences between men and women is the higher incidence of auto-immune disorders encountered by women as exemplified by higher rates of diseases like lupus, rheumatoid arthritis, and multiple sclerosis. These diseases are all related to inflammation. This attack on one's own immune system can also wreck havoc with attempts to regulate metabolism, so crucial in controlling weight and fat metabolism (use and storage).

Possible Liver Taxation

A relatively new area of concern is the problem of fatty liver disease. Dr. Robert Lustig from UCSF, in a series called "The Skinny on Fat," demonizes fructose (fruit sugar) as the prominent culprit in the obesity epidemic and specifically in the abnormal taxation of the liver. Lustig contends, with significant, legitimate academic and scientific support, that since the inception of the pervasive use of HFCS (High Fructose Corn Syrup) in virtually every packaged, processed food that we eat, the incidence of obesity, diabetes, and fatty liver disease has escalated.

Fructose can only be metabolized in the liver and it *must* go through this vital organ every time it is ingested. Dr. Keith Horvath, a cardio-thoracic surgeon from Johns Hopkins Hospital, and his colleagues have determined that obesity "ages" the liver to such an extent that the organ can manifest the properties of someone many years older than the individual in this compromised state. Dr. Lustig calls fructose a "Chronic, dose-dependent liver toxin." Again, low-carb eating wins out in the battle of overweight and health. Behaviorally, it is noted that women do, in fact, appear to be more "addicted" to carbohydrates than men. The hypothesis for this phenomenon is that during hormonal fluctuations, all folks have a more pronounced response to carbohydrates in the pleasure and reward center in the brain. In simple terms, just as in any addictive or "hard to resist" behavior, eating carbs drives a more irresistible state to the stimulant (in this case carbs). It is common knowledge that women encounter more hormonal fluctuations (in number and significance) than men do on a regular basis.

Lower Testosterone

I have observed through the years that quite a few women who are weight-loss resistant have been discovered to have extremely low levels of testosterone production. Yes, women do produce some testosterone and without it they are very hard pressed to achieve ketosis (fat burning metabolism) and to increase lean tissue (muscle and bone) mass and activity. I strongly advise that women having weight-loss problems (especially over 40) have their testosterone levels tested.

I am not an endocrinologist, but my experience working with some of the top individuals in this medical discipline indicates that forward thinking practitioners have begun to routinely prescribe subtle doses of testosterone replacement in women whose blood tests reveal lower than optimal levels. I have seen some significant positive responses, including enhanced weight-loss efforts supported by this expertly applied augmentation.

Behaviorally, it should be noted that high intensity resistance training has been strongly associated with increases in the levels of testosterone secreted in men and women.

Osteoporosis

Osteoporosis may not hinder weight loss, but it is a disease that affects more women than men, so I wanted to address it in this chapter. I have had great success in managing and treating osteoporosis, as I've been told by large numbers of referring physicians.

This disease can be described most simply as a loss of bone mass or density. I have always believed that bones and muscles are intricately connected both in function and physiology. In fact, I have seen the term "bone/muscle unit" mentioned in the scientific literature and have thought that was a helpful description in understanding the relationship and interaction between the two.

I simply understood it as a given that bone density could be influenced directly by muscle stimulation. In my mind there is a simple relationship between muscle growth and bone growth. When observing the patterns of development and degeneration of both bone and muscle mass, the following is obvious: When skeletal muscle is being enhanced or developed, the skeleton is also in a growth phase. When we lose muscle, we lose bone, such as through aging or inactivity. When we gain muscle, we gain bone, such as during puberty, strength training, or hormonal intervention.

It has been my common experience that the women who are most susceptible to osteopenia (the initial phase of bone loss) and osteoporosis (full-fledged bone loss) respond very positively to high intensity resistance training. I have observed the reversal of the trajectory of bone loss occurring as a common response for years. Fortunately, many of my female subjects in this classification have been able to quit using some of the damaging osteoporosis medications.

Here's the simple science: When a modality (exercise in this case) drives protein uptake in the muscle system, the surrounding bones are subject to the same process of building protein content. Structurally, bones are composed of a protein matrix (think of it as a "spider web") upon which the body lays down calcium. The stronger and more integral the protein matrix becomes, the easier it is for it to lay down calcium and the more difficult it becomes to leech that calcium from those bones. Of course, there are nutritional considerations, including adequate calcium consumption and mineral ratios, but they must be included in a process that "drives" the calcium uptake. The simple story: Build muscle/ Build bones.

The Solution for Women? Be SMaRT

As we've discussed, women often do have a more difficult time with weight loss than men for a variety of metabolic and hormonal reasons. Whatever the cause, they will have more success on the SMaRT plan. High intensity exercise counters many of these issues and drives the body toward health.

Ellen was a 45-year-old mother of three. She had always been conscious of her weight but never extremely overweight except after the birth of her third son. She had trained with weights on and off ever since high school, and she was a conscientious runner for quite a few years.

At the time Ellen began her five-week SMaRT program, she was training for marathons and half marathons and was also weight training with a personal trainer. The incorporation of the twice a week SMaRT program replaced Ellen's other weight training, although she continued her running program.

At the end of her five-week metabolic makeover, Ellen lost 30 percent of her existing body fat and increased her strength by more than 25 percent in her upper and lower body. She became as lean as she had been since college, with more muscle than at any time in her life! She has continued her program for the past 10 years and has even added a measurable degree of bone density—no small feat for a gal going from 45 to 55 years of age. Her workouts average about 14 minutes per session, twice a week. She also trains her mother twice a week. Her mom is 80 years old and going strong the SMaRT way!

• • •

In summary, the basic SMaRT program has proven to be highly effective in the majority of cases. Some women do present more difficult, more resistant weight-loss scenarios, in which case the considerations mentioned here might be worth investigating. Besides wanting the ultimate weight-loss solution, many people (women especially) are searching for an anti-aging secret. In chapter nine we'll examine the aging athlete and how our observations of these professional sports players can be applied to the rest of us. Want to know the best anti-aging formula? Keep reading. . . .

CHAPTER 9

THE AGING ATHLETE IN ALL OF US

With the meteoric rise in the number of baby boomers, it occurs to me that the topic of aging athletes might be of significant interest. We are all used to seeing professional athletes extend their careers fruitfully to ages that were heretofore not encountered. In other words, they play longer and at higher levels than was previously common. Much higher levels in the realms of physical capacity and performance level are now widely accepted and even expected of all of us—athletes or not—as we age. So how do we meet these expectations and to what levels can we reasonably aspire? And can the SMaRT program help us remain healthy and strong as we age?

With the increased attention to DNA research, scientists are discovering that some people have different genetic "markers" directly associated with aging. Interestingly, some of these markers have proven to be influenced—quite strongly in some cases—by behavior. In simple terms, that means the activities and habits that you incorporate into your lifestyle plan can affect how you age.

One of my plans in the near future is to get some of my ex-pro-athlete buddies together to help me deliver sensible lifestyle plans, including controlled carb eating and safe and productive high intensity exercise to retired pro athletes. In my mind, these guys (historically, mostly men) have, at one time, led very active lives—including highly demanding physical training—but paid little attention to controlled eating regimens. At this next stage of their noncompetitive lives, they obviously engage in considerably less muscle-building activity, rarely continuing the degree of physically demanding exercise, and commonly do NOT adapt an appropriately controlled eating pattern. With the right program, we can all age better, keep off the weight, and maintain strong, healthy bodies.

Retired Athletes and Weight Gain

Athletes represent baby boomers in an exaggerated manner as a microcosm of what happens to all of us as we get older. Here's the athlete scenario: Young, fit athletes undertake extreme physical tasks, including high intensity (usually high impact, high "force") maneuvers, ostensibly performed to enhance athletic performance potential. Remember, these are young people. It's hard to find a more responsive, more resilient population than young, active folks. Most of us certainly fit into this category at some point of our lives, at least in a relative sense. The majority of us were more active and fit in our twenties than we became in our 40s and 50s, for example.

Take a look at the rookie photos of our professional athletes and compare them with photos of them 10 years later. Even during their active careers in their respective sports, most of them gain significant amounts of weight. Some of that weight gain is actually increased muscle mass accompanied by some smaller degree of fat gain. Almost no pro athlete competes at the same weight at age 30 that they did at age 20. This can most benignly be described as maturation. Now, take a look at the photos of these same guys 10 to 15 years after they retire (many are still relatively "young"). Some are unrecognizably changed! Next, take a look at your college or high school graduation class photos and compare them with 25-year reunion photos. You'll see the same changes as described with the aging athletes.

Why does this happen? What are the metabolic changes that have led to this unfortunate discrepancy? Is it inevitable? To a limited extent, yes, but absolutely NOT at the level and rate that is commonplace. My personal observation is that the most significant change in both appearance and health from younger to older stages is WEIGHT (more specifically, fat mass). The people who maintained fairly consistent body weight through the aging process change the least. In other words, weight gain is the single most contributory characteristic representing aging. Think about it. It's virtually undeniable.

Changes in Body Chemistry and Behavior

The common thread that ages us as time passes is based on our chemistry undergoing fluctuations. However, the degree to which this occurs is significantly dependent upon habits and behavior. For example, it is not uncommon for sex hormones (testosterone, estrogen) and growth hormones (primarily human growth hormone) to decline as time goes by, but both testosterone and human growth hormone levels are stimulated by high intensity exercise.

Another hormone related to aging is that old culprit insulin. While it is true that the beta cells in the pancreas (the ones that secrete insulin) can lose some level of productivity, the management of carbohydrate eating can greatly reduce the workload imposed upon them.

So what have we just described as being strongly correlated to reducing and slowing the chemistry of the aging process? The SMaRT system of eating and exercising: high intensity exercise and controlled carb eating. The logical question is how does a regimen that has historically been so successful at producing fat loss and muscle gain provide such a strong "anti-aging" effect? Keep reading....

What Can We Learn from Aging Athletes?

Back to the aging athlete analogy: When athletes become less active and perhaps cease to train and compete at a high demand level, they simply represent the more gradual aging process in all of us at an accelerated rate. In a way, athletes remind me of animals that have a much shorter life span than humans. We get to witness longer term metabolic processes occur in much shorter time frames than is normally encountered, and we can learn valuable lessons from the study of these patterns.

Here is an assumption I have made with a few others who have some background in insulin-resistant-related health problems. All hormones have functions and are part of a chemical balancing act we like to call health. It is when these powerful signaling proteins (hormones) become imbalanced that health and functional problems ensue. Insulin is one major player in this scenario. We have reviewed the concept that overproduction of insulin occurs when the receptors of this chemical become inefficient due to overload of carbohydrate eating and/or the constant presence of high levels of insulin in the bloodstream and simply become "worn out."

As young, strong individuals, athletes who are slightly insulin resistant might be at an advantage in certain sports. This is not a highly reviewed concept, but it seems that the upside of some insulin resistant tendencies might be increased energy storage and muscle building in young athletes. Remember, at prime athletic ages and engaging at intense levels of physical exertion, the presence of high insulin levels can be well managed and balanced by high levels of hormones, such as human growth hormone and testosterone. In simple terms, the hormone status that might be highly advantageous for young athletes might be a double-edged sword as they age, promoting some disadvantageous health circumstances, including weight gain and prediabetic tendencies.

We quite commonly observe the physical appearance of many of our iconic athletes change overnight. While it would seem reasonable that some subtle changes would occur as a result of normal aging, the speed and severity of the physical decline of some of these athletes is both remarkable and disturbing. I would propose that the situation can be readily diagnosed and easily reversed.

The basic problem with the aging athlete acutely—and all of us a little more gradually as we enter our 40s and beyond—is that we are generally unaware of the subtle changes that occur metabolically in an exaggerated fashion to athletes and at a more modest but similarly pervasive rate in the general population. The simple explanation is that our metabolic rate slows down.

SMaRT Aging

What is the nature of these changes and how can we learn from observing the rapid decline in our sports heroes? Perhaps the answer to why we have changes that affect our body's direction in this aging process lies in some of our behaviors that DON'T change. In other words, the question arises as to whether aging is an inevitable, chronological degeneration or a culmination of lifelong behaviors that direct the rate of aging.

Since aging competitive athletes engage in much less higher intensity muscle work, they normally lose significant volumes of muscle mass. That means that the body is demanding energy at an exceedingly reduced rate 24 hours a day. Why is that important? Because non-resting (active) metabolism uses only about 30 percent of total calories, and the generation of body heat requires only about 10 percent of calories. The other 60 percent of burned calories comes from your resting metabolic rate. That's why one of our main goals in the Metabolic Makeover program is the increase in muscle mass and activity.

The most likely answer to the inevitable versus the controllable character of aging is that both of these factors probably have some influence on the final outcome. Volumes of clinical data and study analysis do indicate that engagement in vigorous exercise and disciplined eating both (separately and combined) provide powerful anti-aging properties to one's lifestyle.

The key topic is commonly referred to as "anti-aging." Simply stated, people don't want to be subjected to the chronological aging process so regularly accepted as inevitable. Well, as a simple observation of modern behavior, people will go to great and in many cases expensive lengths to combat the signs of aging. How about this novel concept? Keep your body from degenerating metabolically. What does that mean? How does that translate into action?

Let's examine the physiological differences between young people and older people. The following are my observations over many years of clinical practice and an extensive review of scientific literature related to the subject: I would rate the state of the circulatory system as the number one differentiator between young and old. Ask any surgeon's opinion regarding the difference between dealing with young and old patients and they will tell you that it is best represented by the difference in young and old blood vessels.

With regard to a healthy circulatory system, traditionally high intensity exercise instigates a decrease in total cholesterol, and there is a strong improvement in cholesterol composition. Harmful LDL cholesterol levels decrease slightly, and HDL cholesterol levels rise significantly. Together, these changes produce a strong reduction—meaning improvement—in the atherogenic index. The atherogenic index is simply a measurement of blood vessel health.

This makes all the sense in the world because the circulatory system delivers the energy that each functioning cell relies upon so critically. The circulatory system supports the precious functional level of the heart. The great news for followers of the SMaRT system is that the invigorator and instigator of optimal circulatory health is the MUSCLE system. More good news: A major impediment to youthful circulatory function is "glycation," which, in simplified terms, means "sugar-ication." The takeaway is that controlled carb eating provides less sugar to be metabolized and handled by the blood vessels and therefore contributes heavily to a more youthful circulatory functional status.

Next in importance in the aging process is the metabolic rate or vitality of your body chemistry. Again, the most substantial stimulator of youthful metabolic activity is the state of the muscle system. Nothing short of drastic pharmaceutical intervention can affect metabolic status more than the muscle-building stimulus derived from high intensity exercise.

Mental attitude, in my opinion, is another critical component as it relates to any health or performance evaluation. Younger people are noticeably more upbeat traditionally than older folks. Some of this may be behavioral since younger individuals are less likely to have faced negative or failed scenarios than their older counterparts. On the other hand, some of this might certainly be attributable to the hormone status of younger folks. However, all of us have experienced the absolute delight of being in the presence of older people who have great, vigorous attitudes and energy levels that defy their chronological age and inspire all of us.

My friend Sy is a great example of exactly how the SMaRT program works so well as we age. I've known Sy for more than 30 years, and I used to play golf with him occasionally. He was always gregarious, happy go lucky, and *fat*. Fast forward 25 years: I hadn't seen him for about 20 years, but I heard his voice in a small fitness center in Coronado, California. I knew it was him. He looked better (having lost some weight) and was in the gym (all good news). I showed him how to move slowly when training with weights, and he could feel the difference immediately. He was 84 years old at the time.

The next summer I finally saw Sy again. He was shuffling along, head down and quiet. I thought perhaps he had had a stroke. When I asked him what happened, he said he was diagnosed with some slipped discs four months earlier. I asked him what he was doing for it. He told me the doctors told him to rest and take it easy. I told him that was the dumbest thing I'd ever heard!

Sy said he was going to have to quit his golf club. He had been a member for 35 years and loved going there and playing with the boys.

I said, "No you're not! I'm going to work with you," and I promised him that in three weeks we would be hitting golf balls together.

He said I was crazy.

Starting that day I had him stretch mildly and begin a SMaRT resistance program for his whole body. I knew that it would be safe and simple enough for him to perform—even with his slipped discs—and that it would be an efficient way for him to effectively achieve better health. He called me the next day and said he actually felt better than he had in four months! Three weeks later we went to the driving range and hit golf balls together. Within four months he was doing high intensity training twice a week. His workout takes about 16 minutes, but he stays at the fitness center for about two hours, holding court with anyone who enters. He got down to 13 percent body fat and does a workout that would tax a well-conditioned 40-year-old. He's past 87 now and shows his muscles to everyone, saying he feels like a tiger!

• • •

I have witnessed hundreds of people who have seemingly reversed the clock by incorporating the behaviors that I have presented in this book. Many of these folks literally look five, ten, or even more years younger than they did at the inception of the SMaRT undertaking. You will be surprised to experience the noticeable difference in the way you feel, look, and act once you've attained the next level (or two) of fitness and health that is yours for the taking, when you follow the advice provided in this book.

Have we discovered the fountain of youth? Probably not, but it's as close as we can get at this point in time. Stay youthful and prosper...be SMaRT!

CHAPTER 10

TIPS FOR TRAINERS

Many people think of me as a trainer, since I do take on a small number of patients and clients for personal programs. However, I have always considered myself a teacher and clinician in the application of exercise as a health and performance modality. When I first started my practice in the early 1970s, there was really no such thing as personal training. In fact, my most productive operation took place in the 1980s, when my Nautilus facility ran up to 35 people an hour through their SMaRT training regimens, with five instructors on the floor using four interchangeable circuits of equipment. Believe me, everyone received personal attention when it mattered, at the critical points of each set, and people encouraged each other to reach their limits and objectives.

I always personally took on special referral cases from doctors and therapists and worked very closely with some great sports/medicine professionals. We all had genuine respect for each other's roles in the treatment and health processes of our charges.

I continue to get most of my trainees from referrals and have never done any advertising for business. In fact, you can't *join* my facility. My facility does personal services programs: personal training, corporate programs, rehab programs, and study projects so there are no actual traditional "members" to join the center. Each year the insurance company sends an inspector to see what's going on in the facilities they insure to ascertain if they're up to professional standards. One year the insurance fellow came and I was the only one in my center in the middle of the afternoon. He asked me how many members I had. I said, "Four." He asked me how many years I'd been in business. I said, "Forty." He asked why there weren't any more people coming to my facility. I told him that "I liked to keep it private." What I didn't tell him is that we only do individual programs and have no official membership status for anyone. I'm sure he left shaking his head, probably thinking I was some Italian mob guy from New York, running some fitness center cover scam.

My facilities are intentionally never crowded and always set up to accommodate the people who are training there. In fact, I always leave plenty of open time to run IRB studies, wherein we may have to handle up to 100 "extra" people for 5 to 12 weeks at a time. IRB studies are controlled, overseen studies that conform to professional standards of care and objectivity as determined by an outside board. Another famous Dr. Ben line I use is that my places are so exclusive that we don't want *anybody* to use them! That usually gets 'em!

Whenever I go to a commercial or public fitness center to work out, I am constantly amazed at the absolutely useless workouts I see taking place around me. After all these years, it never ceases to amaze me that folks commonly do the same senseless crap that they were doing 50 years ago. "Going through the motions" would be the most charitable way to describe the gyrations I routinely witness.

It seems critical to me that this genre of personal trainers be addressed for the good of the discipline of exercise and the folks that participate and put themselves in the hands of these professionals. A number of certification operations exist, but in my experience the subjects of exercise history, simple science, and helpful application of this information for the trainers seem lacking in the field.

I have had hundreds of trainers come to me for help over the years. Unfortunately, they have already completed their required studies and often admit to me that they learn more in two weeks working in my facilities with myself and my staff than they did in months and in some cases, years, of formal study. Common example: I saw a "certified" trainer putting some older gals (probably younger than I am) through a routine for some unidentifiable purpose. The reason I criticize the exercises is that they seemed disconnected and lacking in specific purpose (like squatting while doing overhead presses in the same movement). Why complicate the endeavor and detract value from each of these exercises? As a result, I have two major problems and questions with that scenario: one, certified for what, by whom? What was the program content of the certification? How did the trainer demonstrate proficiency?

And two: What was the purpose or main objective of the routine or regimen that was provided? In my opinion the construction of "exercise" regimens is subject to whim, trends, "new discoveries" in supposed science, and the simple case of this year's new models (just like cars). The old stuff can't work as well as the new stuff, can it? Strengthen the core, train functionally, "fast twitch" muscle training, and more cryptic descriptions of variations on silly themes are the recycled, "new" ideas in fitness.

It seems to me that there are so many "specialists" in the fields of exercise, training, and therapy that very few can provide a simply designed, productive routine of exercise that meets the basic needs of the client or patient. People don't need a battery of tests run to determine that they are too fat, too weak, and lack the energy necessary to muster a healthy and productive lifestyle. That's what most folks want and what we, as professionals, should be driven to achieve with them.

The two most prominent and productive behaviors that can contribute most significantly to the needs and aspirations of the overwhelming majority of our population are exercise and diet. If we could make it a serious goal to have all Americans who need to lose at least 10 pounds of fat, lose it and increase their overall body strength by 25 percent, we could alleviate a huge percentage of our health problems and probably reduce our medical expenses by at least 50 percent! Neither of these goals is exceptionally difficult to attain given the information we now hold and the simple methods described in this book. Let's get going!

The Art of Exercise Training

If human performance was so cut and dried, we could simply use a computer, create an algorithm, and progressively program exercise sessions up to some perfectly predictable path of continuously higher levels of fitness and health. Sorry, it doesn't work that way! One of the most compelling reasons that the SMaRT approach works so well is that it is utterly subjective and pliable. You simply can't preordain that someone's next exercise session should be constructed exactly, based upon the previous session, because there are too many variables.

Here's how I explain human performance: A person sets a world record in an event one week. The next week that person comes in fifth in the same event. What happened? Life happened! The dynamics of physiology happened! Remember when we talked about health being a dynamic, ever-changing process? Well, each exercise session is influenced by an enormous set of variables every time we engage in one. How did you sleep the night before? How well can you concentrate today? What are you hormone levels, your enzyme balances, your fuel availabilities, and so on? That's why no one can tell you how many repetitions you should do in each exercise. That's pure nonsense!

For example, when training a client, in each set, what was the "load" time of each rep? How much did the exerciser accentuate the negative aspect of each rep? How well did he or she maintain proper posture? How focused was the trainee? How hard could he or she "push" that day? The combination of variables is almost infinite! Each exercise training session is an event constructed based on a general blueprint with the final detail to be determined during the actual performance of that session.

Know Your Client

Each trainer's job is to get the most out of their clients each time they work with them. Here's what you can do to get the most out of each trainee, each time. Know your discipline—the science and application of anatomy and physiology. Pay attention, and know your client. People ask me if I ever get tired of doing the same thing over and over for all these years. My reply is that it might be the thousandth time I'm doing something, but it might be the first time that that person actually *gets* some critical point or *feels* a specific muscle controlling the movement. That's new territory for them and real progress in the process.

Each session is an opportunity to make some little change in that person's health and well-being. First, ascertain the objectives of the trainee. What is it that he or she is trying to accomplish? This seems simplistic, but many folks can't really organize and verbalize their intentions or at least aspirations without some guidance and directed questioning. Once the trainer has established the agreed-upon objectives, by trainer and trainee, design a regimen of exercise and eating that will most efficiently and effectively drive the associated responses. This is *not* as complicated as it might appear on the surface. Throughout my long career, I have noted an absolute universality of fitness and health objectives. Everyone wants to attain a leaner, stronger, more highly functionally capable physiology and appearance. I can't put a definite number on it, but I would suggest that those aspirations include the overwhelming majority of prospective trainees. Finally, the health and fitness plan should be constructed and applied with these goals in mind: safety, efficiency, productivity, and long-term adherence.

Safety

No one can rationalize exposing exercisers to higher risk movements when lower risk options are available and superior drivers of progress! However, the industry is inundated with obviously rigorous "high energy" regimens that promise exceptional levels of fitness, leanness, and so on, as verified by humorously presented (at least to me) models of success. Desperate people will buy anything, but we have all witnessed the enormous drop-out rate of these programs. To reiterate: Any programs that people don't do because they are injured, or won't do because the routines are just too obligatory and taxing, are useless. The tease of training like a Navy Seal or an elite athlete should be so irrelevant to most of the population that it could be defined as delusional. It's just part of the bait offered to the uneducated public. One of the major goals of this book is to educate!

It has been established recently that high intensity exercise, applied prudently, is capable of inducing superior benefits to all populations. However, as I have touched upon previously, the topic is misunderstood and misapplied in most cases. I think I have established, through the last 40 years of successful application, that high intensity exercise can be safe and highly productive for every stratum of fitness level.

Safety never has to be compromised in order to deliver highly effective exercise. As an additional caveat, nutritional education and advice should also follow the tenets of safety. Here is where the trainer or fitness advisor has a more precarious situation. The current state of affairs drives stagnation with regard to nutritional science. As a result, the advice that one is given "permission" to disseminate (by whom, no one really knows!) is limited, severely outdated, and apparently harmful on a large scale.

How can I make such a sweeping claim? Here's how: Since the preponderance of our national nutritional concerns have been dominated by the demonization of dietary fat regarding its "association" with obesity, diabetes etc., for the past 50 years, how could ANYONE imagine that this obsession has proven to be anything but harmful? It hasn't helped. We've gone—and continue to go—backwards!

So here's how I handle this dilemma and advise my practitioners to handle it. Explain to your trainees that your experience and study have led you to the tenets you suggest they follow. I also advise patients, clients, and subjects of studies to read some relevant books, articles, and research papers that might provide a corresponding philosophy and even material from the "other" side or, as our friend Darth would say, The Dark Side.

There should be no hidden agenda found in this book. The facts and opinions are presented as such. Simple carbohydrates and sugars have proven to be the bane of our modern eating habits. The fear of fat philosophy has compounded the issue and yet some unidentified power wants only "professionals" to provide nutritional information. Who *are* these folks? MDs? Registered dieticians? That would be great except for the reality that MDs will readily admit that they have no formal training in nutrition. And who has access to registered dieticians? To compound the issue, dieticians have to follow doctor's orders, in many cases, so it's the blind leading the blind.

Perhaps more problematic, other "nutritionists" (there are many programs out there that allow people to call themselves nutritionists after very little course work as opposed to registered dieticians who do complete a much more rigorous and substantial academic curriculum) generally have no oversight and that's usually not good for the consumer or patient.

In many cases, government-issued ideas are relied upon as the basis for solid, reliable, and objective nutritional dogma. I hope I have adequately conveyed the point that government health advice has a very poor track record. Unfortunately, the big industry influences in the fields of health and specifically nutrition upon government's philosophies can't help but skew the advice away from objectivity and helpful logic!

So my final advice to trainers and exercise leaders is to suggest that their philosophy is what they conclude is best for themselves and their families and explain how they came to this conclusion. There is plenty of ammunition, in this book, to mount a logical and scientifically sound stance on the subject.

Efficiency

No one I've encountered in my almost 50 years of exercise and fitness experience wants to waste any time or effort in the process of becoming healthy and fit! It follows logically that any trainer who can drive consistent, positive benefits for his/her clients will be successful—especially if their program offers a palatable time commitment.

The entire functional and physiological basis for the SMaRT program is based upon this vital tenet—efficiency. We simply must, as a nation, uncover a potent, consistent solution to sedentary behavior and metabolic degeneration. At this point in time, no more consistently beneficial exercise regimen exists, providing the highest rate of return for effort, than the SMaRT program.

In practical terms, trainers and trainees can "get the job done" in 15 to 20 minutes, twice per week. The client is in and out in record time, leaving satisfied that they have fulfilled their requirement for optimally effective exercise. The trainer can handle a higher volume of clients per unit of time and the facility can service more satisfied customers each day. There is no downside in a theoretical or practical sense.

Lastly, on a physiological, scientific note, efficiency of physical effort has everything to do with long-term adherence and eventual success for each of that system's followers. Trainers, I urge you to use common sense and have the confidence that good science must always dictate the parameters of any rational exercise program.

Productivity

At this point we have established that safety and efficiency are vital components of a successful fitness and health plan. However, the bottom line in any program for any purpose is productivity. What is the level of progress accomplished by the application of our plans? In simple terms, does it work?

If it does work, then the participants will, in most scenarios, lose body fat, increase lean tissue, and correspondingly increase metabolic rate. In addition, you can expect that decreases in resting blood pressure, heart rate, triglycerides, and inflammatory factors will follow. Strength and endurance levels should increase as well as a sense of well-being and energy, perhaps even a notable elevation of mood and motivational status. All of these effects have been measured and reported in the scientific literature and should be known and referred to by the trainer as support for the legitimacy of the program.

Of course, responses to any intervention vary with the individual, but as a general course of events, the aforementioned indices of progress should be part and parcel of any productive plan.

Long-term Adherence

If we can agree that exercise is an integral part of a sensible fitness and health program, then it makes perfect sense that the participant should adopt this behavior on a lifelong, continuous basis. Remember, no medicine can work if we don't take it! The elements suggested—safety, efficiency, and productivity—are the basis for long-term program adherence. If the trainee never gets hurt, spends a minimum of time, and achieves success, it is much more likely that he or she will include this behavior in his or her regularly scheduled events.

The SMaRT system has something I've never noted in any other program: people who have endorsed and practiced it for twenty, thirty, and even forty years successfully and consistently. I find that extremely powerful and personally rewarding!

The Strength Curve versus Resistance Curve

There are a few elements that elevate an exercise session from the mundane to a potentially productive and meaningful experience. The following concepts have not been discussed by anyone in the field. For all the significance that some of the exercise training systems profess, none have enunciated nor have they demonstrated any cognition of the existence of these. Strength curve versus resistance curve: A critical acknowledgement of optimal performance when supervising resistance training, especially slow resistance training, is the dichotomy between the trainee's strength curve and the resistance curve provided by the resistance device.

Trainers should know this, but in many cases, they don't. The resistance curve of an exercise device can be defined as the variation of torque or applicable counterforce plotted throughout the exercise range. For example, if a bicep curl machine provided 10-foot pounds of torque at the starting position, 20-foot pounds at 90 degrees, and then 10 again at the end position, then those points plotted on a graph would configure a "curve" representing the change in effective resistance. That's the resistance curve.

The strength curve of an exerciser can be defined as the variation in demonstrable strength potential throughout the exercise range. For example, during a bicep curl, the trainee is capable of producing 20-foot pounds of torque at the beginning, 20 at mid-range, and 10 at the end position. Those points plotted on a graph would configure a much different "curve" than the curve produced by the aforementioned machine's plotted resistance curve.

The difference between the two curves, the resistance curve of the machine and the strength curve of the trainee, are different. They are NOT the same, actually and proportionately. So what does all this mean in real life? It means that some designs of machines are more accommodating than others and NONE can be "perfect" for anyone in a mechanical sense nor could any devotee or designer of any exercise device presume a perfect match for everyone. That's just foolish and silly, but there *is* something we can do to approach a better marriage between the resistance curve and the strength curve.

I'm a bit surprised and rather disappointed that no other "master" trainer or "founder" of any slow exercise cult has broached this subject. I suspect that they are seriously lacking in the interpretation of the subtleties of resistance training. From my experience, I have consistently noted an absence of the recognition of the many influential components of successful exercise.

Trainers, please try to grasp the following concept: If you have explained the points of constant load, focus, and an acceptable, controlled technique, and your trainee has adopted these elements into his/her performance, it then follows that the demonstration of the trainee's strength curve as it relates to the resistance curve of the device involved will be obviously manifested. Please, read that again. It is a mouthful and I'll explain this subtle, important concept. At that point (and ANY point) in the exercise movement, when the resistance curve and the strength curve bifurcate or don't "match up," the attentive trainee will demonstrate that differentiation. If the resistance curve becomes relatively, albeit momentarily, overwhelming, your trainee will compensate by changing speed, posture, or obvious effort—or some combination of these.

In my world and under my construction of slow resistance techniques, this is not only acceptable but also diagnostically helpful. These "adjustments" indicate an advanced recognition by the trainer and the trainee that this system of exercise is dynamic and human, not static and mechanistic as some have proposed. The bottom line is that the intensity and consistency of loading are successfully maintained while these technique adjustments are applied.

Think about this: If you were to allow "perfect" form during a repetition by reducing the load to a point wherein the most divergent point between the resistance curve and the strength curve was a "non-issue," then it is likely that that same resistance is inadequate for much of the rest of the range of motion. This is an extremely subtle concept and has, to my knowledge, never been broached by any other contributor, expert or not, in the field.

With regard to the diagnostic value of slow training, the following should be noted: One of the unintended benefits of this style of exercising that I developed is the absence of the "white noise" that explosive or conventionally rapid, rhythmical repetition systems create. It is in this controlled pace of movement that the subtleties and aberrations of demonstrable strength can be readily assessed. I cannot tell you how many problematic conditions I have discovered by the simple observation of difficulties encountered by trainees who demonstrate an inability to perform a movement comfortably or symmetrically. One of the great advantages of moving very slowly during exercise movements is that one is able to diagnose specifically what exact position in that movement is problematic. We are able to pinpoint that position because we are not simply rushing by any one position and are more cognizant and "connected" to the precision of each segment of each repetition. The first option is to work "around" the deficit and if it continues to be problematic, a referral to a diagnostic practitioner is usually mandated. If a trainer develops a solid, professional reputation, a good working relationship can be created with the appropriate medical and health providers. This is an invaluable situation for the trainer and wonderful for his/her clients.

Personalization

Since this profession that many people practice is called "personal" training, it might behoove us to deal with the subject of personalization to some extent. This is the basis of another bone I have to pick with the behavior reported to me about some of the slow-training renegades. The absence of personality or interaction with clients is an element I lament. It is NOT necessary to be officiously professional in order to convey professional competence. The folks you're working with are commonly fairly well-educated and concerned with their health and fitness. The trainer has a wonderful opportunity to interact on a personal and professional level with some very worthwhile people. My best advice is to provide an educated, well-planned program with which you have a comfortable level of expertise and confidence with regard to authenticity. People can pick up on bluster and company lines. Know your discipline and know your clients.

In a practical sense, there is a huge difference between being personable and presenting a vacuous stream of chatter. It's perfectly reasonable to become friendly with people you're working with. After all, you are both working towards a mutually rewarding end—that of enhanced fitness, health, and overall well-being. Be encouraging and be honest with your charges. When the time comes to demand effort, don't be shy but always be positive. We have to expect that these folks are paying you and showing up because they want to succeed. I often tell people that "I'm an entertaining guy but I'm not here to entertain them." My job and yours is to apply our knowledge earnestly and personably to these good folks. There is no need to be distant and feign some ultra professionalism as some slow systems advocate. That's just nonsense and serves to debase the interaction to the point of an obviously super-cilious endeavor.

Another unintended benefit of slow training is that the ele-ments of any set of exercise can be broken down succinctly into three phases: the setup, the continuation, and the "all out drive to the fin-ish." Each of these phases can exist for anywhere from ten seconds to no more than thirty seconds, in almost every case. If you as the trainer can recognize these designations, you can verbally guide the trainee to a significantly higher level of focus and performance. This is advanced material, but it can make a real difference if you can time the communication and reinforcement of these delineated segments. This interaction provides the ultimate personalization and the opti-mally applied understanding of the process!

Training Athletes

I started off in the field of exercise and performance as a competi-tive athlete. The preparation for these endeavors fascinated me from the very start (Little League 1965 World Champions: Mid Island, Staten Island, NY). We hit it, training in earnest to pre-pare for the World Championships, and I thought it was "cool" to be pushed to the limit. The tricky part about training any athlete is that you're dealing with a process that is 60 percent psychological, 20 percent cerebral, and maybe 20 percent physical. Usually, you're dealing with folks who have special wiring (sometimes "loose wir-ing"). I know because I was one of them. It is therefore, in my experi-ence, incumbent upon anyone working with athletes to understand the special circumstances of the process.

Athletic prowess and performance are not necessarily related to any health protection status. In simple terms, the fact that some-one can run a marathon in two-and-a-half hours instead of three-and-a-half hours does not correlate with any higher level of *health*. Yes, people who exercise more are statistically healthier than those who exercise less. That is a perfect example of association rather than causation.

There are two separate areas of preparation for all athletes in any sport: conditioning (general) and sport performance (specific). There are quite a few books dedicated to each major sport, many of them written by acknowledged sports stars. However, I found that the ones I've been exposed to are simplistic or simply regurgitations of standard fare. The exercise books that spin off into sports training advisements or at least chapters dedicated to specific sports training seem bizarre to me. I have often thought that these authors must have never played the particular sport for which they provide programs. In my opinion, exercise "experts" should stick to their own discipline, rather than provide the biased input that some tweak in their basic system meets the demands of sports specific training. Professionals would be well advised that ALL human (athletic) performance is propelled by enhancing *general* potential (strength, flexibility, endurance) and then developing *specific* skills that apply uniquely to that particular event. As a professional trainer, one should be required to understand the basic elements of athletic performance and then attempt to develop some sub-specialization with additional training and hands-on coaching internships.

All athletes would stand to gain considerably by the application of a basic conditioning program designed to efficiently enhance muscle strength, cardiovascular endurance, and basic flexibility safely with a *minimal* time commitment. That really does describe the organizational constructs of the SMaRT plan. What it does NOT mean is that the SMaRT plan should be considered a complete training program for the preparation of any high-level sports performance.

So here's what I have recommended successfully for athletes: Engage in a basic conditioning program to develop a functional base for performance. Spend the bulk of the training time doing those maneuvers (skill, drills, and so on) that will be applied specifically in the sports performance. Pitchers have to pitch; football linemen have to drive off the ball; basketball players have to shoot, shuffle, jump, and reach for the ball. So pitchers should throw and work on the fine, specific techniques involved. Linemen have to drive from a crouched position, and basketball players have to practice the specific movements of shooting, rebounding, and playing defense, and so on.

A word of warning from years of firsthand experience: Trends in the realm of training athletes are very powerful. Without mentioning names, I worked with some high-profile strength coaches and trainers of professional teams. When their teams were winning, everyone wanted to emulate their systems and be taught by them. When, a few years later, these same professionals with the exact same programs were associated with losing teams, their advice was quickly disavowed and the next winning team's systems became the newest and greatest trend in the training of athletes. Know the basic science and apply these principles soundly, assessing success by measurable enhanced levels of play and reduced levels of injury.

• • •

I think trainers should take professional and personal pride in what they do. Be responsible and appreciative. You are incredibly lucky to be able to do what you love for a living. Most of the work environments that you perform in are relaxed, friendly, and professional. People come to you voluntarily and pay you because they choose to do so. They are depending on you to guide and encourage them to attain their goals. Enjoy the process and do the best job that you can. Many people—and perhaps the entire nation—are depending on you to turn the situation around and lead them away from poor health and weight gain and toward a lean, fit, healthy, and strong body.

CONCLUSION

People who are active achieve better results—both in exercise and diet—than folks who are not. As has been presented in this book, activity and exercise are two separate and distinct endeavors, but I noted the active advantage long before I made the distinction. Our bodies were designed to need exercise to survive, and the SMaRT program was designed with this in mind.

In terms of diet and nutrition, people who cut calories are primarily cutting carbs, since most people eat the majority of their calories from carbohydrate sources. Given this fact, I believe that the cutting of carbs rather than the cutting of total calories is what actually propels weight loss. Additionally, it has been my experience that the controlling of carbs allows a higher likelihood of long-term success.

Many people who eat the same things quite frequently have a better chance of long-term weight control. If the foods you eat are satisfying and you simply like them, they are easier to stick with as your main staples. I know people who eat chicken five days a week and others who love tuna salad for breakfast and lunch.

Trying to "grind" away calories with huge bouts of exercise is a low percentage endeavor. Think again about how much exercise work it takes to offset two cookies. As a short-term plan, and with strong will power or compulsion, it can work, but in the long run it usually makes you frustrated and cranky. High intensity exercise as performed in the SMaRT plan is what really works when you are trying to lose that stubborn fat.

Those who make repeated efforts at fitness, weight control, and health habits are more likely to achieve some semblance of long-term success. They simply don't give up. Remember that health and fitness are dynamic animals. They are constantly vacillating and always subject to acute and chronic variations. I consider my own health an experiment (in science fiction). It's a challenge but, at the same time, fascinating and enjoyable.

I can recount thousands of cases of seemingly miraculous changes made by seemingly ordinary folks using the principles espoused in this book. The journey provides many rewards despite the ultimate destination.

Never give up.

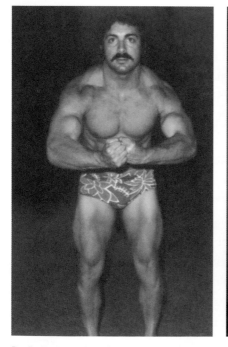 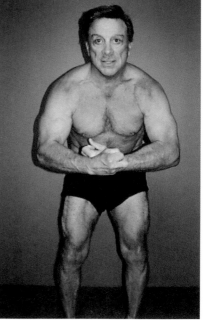

Dr. Ben at age 25 with 6 percent body fat   Dr. Ben at age 65+ with 7 percent body fat

ACKNOWLEDGMENTS

My new family: Ellie, who has helped me get through my technical limitations numerous times. Matt, St. Scottie, and Nick, my "boys." Bob and Evie, who have adopted me as part of the family. The Adams Sisters. Jimmy Speros and family: We have been brothers for many years including all family members from young to old. With little family left, they have been there for all events and circumstances. Til death do us part!

J.B. (John Bass) my Arizona brother. We've solved most of the world's problems together, and Ben and Bridget, my nephew and niece. We've had many great "events" together. Colene and Barry Fernando, always there together through thick and thin. Dick Lund, my brother from another mother. We share the same twisted sense of life and humor. Chuckie, Billy O. Stevie B. Teelie, Markie, Jamie, all part of my extended family since the beginning of the Arizona phase. Warren S. and Lyle B. for 24th St. and Bretski and Sarah Boo-Boo my "gym kids."

Danno and Garootz with me, the "Three Stooges of Golf." Hundreds of amazing stories and laughs. Hoping for many more years of lunacy!

R.D. (Ron Donlick). We've been joined at the hip for more than 50 years. Too many unbelievable stories to tell! Mikey Minardo, the protégé I'm most proud of. A wonderful professional and great friend since he was 13 years old.

No man is successful without a good women in the picture. I have been blessed for the last 50 years with four great loves and soul mates, Judy, Cathy, Tinsi, and Ellie. No man should be so lucky!

Professional friends: Fred Hahn (Atilla the "Hahn"): A great friend and student of the art and science of exercise. If I go to war over slow resistance training, Fred would be my wartime consigliere. Kevin Fontaine: Without a doubt the most practical, high caliber researcher in the field displaying expertise at an unparalleled level. If I'm doing research, Kevin will be involved.

I don't know Doug McGuff, never spoke to him and I suspect that we don't see eye to eye on the application of high intensity principals but, in my opinion, no one has demonstrated a better understanding of the physiology of high intensity exercise. Great work!

Gary Taubes, a friend, cohort and mentor. Can't say enough about his contribution to our fields . . . life-changing work! Peter Attia, great mind demonstrating absolute scientific objectivity. Also does a mean, high level work out. The real deal. The Nusi project they started will provide enormous benefit to the cause of objectivity and legitimate science.

The Sports Conditioning/ Courts of Appeal group: Gary F.—world's strictest trainer, Pat O., Mikey Cuz (the best), Max W, Nicky V, Bob M, Mark S., Tommy D., Stevie A, John A, and Lisa B, . The Tennis crowd: Mike and Greg Hanson, Andy Levison, Hector Munoz, Bobby Andersen, Tony Ameduri, Joe Leopardi, Claude Schoenlank (a "real" tennis player), Jim Barton, Mike Reilly, and many more.

The I.C. players: Spider (Bob Coran), Roach (Ed Rudman), Judy Allen, Ann Chipman, Jackie Lewis, Mixie (Gary Mix), Freddie Recchio, Mike Podlucky,

Freddie Gray, Kenny Wilpon, Steve Long, Mark Sherman, Joel Bonamo, and Ira Reiter and Luga P. . . . great pros and lifelong friends.

Morrow St. Boys . . . Big Nicky, Lenny (God rest him), Pat C., and Richie P. The best partners anyone could ask for . . . solid, honest, great guys.

My cousin Richie T., an accomplished author and indispensable resource and advisor on this book . . . Always a good kid! Cousin Judy—my Mom's favorite.

Lara Asher, my editor. Now I know why people need editors . . . what a talent and a wonderfully nice lady! Hope we can work together again.

My agent Carol Mann. No one has ever been luckier in the book business than I was to somehow get Carol to take on this project. I absolutely hit the jackpot and I know it. I am very grateful for her guidance.

SelectBooks (Sugiharas)—thanks for believing in the project.

For all the people who took my advice and put their health and fitness in my hands, I am forever grateful. I am proud that I always gave my best with no reservation.

RESOURCES/BIBLIOGRAPHY

INTRODUCTION

1. Deaths: Leading Causes for 2012 by Melonie Heron, Ph.D., Division of Vital Statistics.

2. Economic Costs of Diabetes in the U.S. in 2012 2625 Diabetes Care April 2013 vol. 36 no. 4 1033-1046.

3. National Vital Statistics Reports Volume 64, Number 10 August 31, 2015.

4. Prevalence of Childhood and Adult Obesity in the United States, 2011-2012 FREE Cynthia L. Ogden, PhD; Margaret D. Carroll, MSPH; Brian K. Kit, MD, MPH; Katherine M. Flegal, PhD JAMA 2014; 311(8):806-814.

5. The economics of obesity: dietary energy density and energy cost, From the Nutritional Sciences Program, School of Public Health and Community Medicine, University of Washington, Seattle, WA (AD), and Unité 557, Institut National de la Santé et de la Recherche Médicale, Conservatoire National des Arts et Métiers, Institut Scientifique et Technique de la Nutrition et de l'Alimentation, Paris, France (ND). Presented at the symposium "Science-Based Solutions to Obesity: What Are the Roles of Academia, Government, Industry, and Health Care?", held in Boston, MA, March 10–11, 2004 and Anaheim, CA, October 2, 2004. Supported in part by the National Research Initiative of the USDA Cooperative State Research Education and Extension Service grant 2004-35215-14441.

CHAPTER ONE: Evolution and Science

1. Abramson JL and Vaccarino V. Relationship between physical activity and inflammation among apparently healthy middle-aged and older US adults. Arch Intern Med 162: 1286–1292, 2002.

2. Akira S, Taga T, and Kishimoto T. Interleukin-6 in biology and medicine. Adv Immunol 54: 1–78, 1993.

3. Ballou SP, Lozanski FB, Hodder S, Rzewnicki DL, Mion LC, Sipe JD, Ford AB, and Kushner I. Quantitative and qualitative alterations of acute-phase proteins in healthy elderly persons. Age Ageing 25: 224–230, 1996.

4. Barzilay JI, Abraham L, Heckbert SR, Cushman M, Kuller LH, Resnick HE, and Tracy RP. The relation of markers of inflammation to the development of glucose disorders in the elderly: the Cardiovascular Health Study. Diabetes 50: 2384–2389, 2001.

5. Bastard JP, Maachi M, Van Nhieu JT, Jardel C, Bruckert E, Grimaldi A, Robert JJ, Capeau J, and Hainque B. Adipose tissue IL-6 content correlates with resistance to insulin activation of glucose uptake both in vivo and in vitro. J Clin Endocrinol Metab 87: 2084–2089, 2002.

6. Blair SN, Cheng Y, and Holder JS. Is physical activity or physical fitness more important in defining health benefits? Med Sci Sports Exerc 33: S379–S399, 2001.

7. Invited Review 1158 ANTI-INFLAMMATION AND EXERCISE J Appl Physiol • VOL 98 • APRIL 2005.

8. Hellerstein, M. De novo lipogenesis in humans: metabolic and regulatory aspects. National Center for Biotechnology Information. Retrieved August 13, 2014.

9. Borghouts, L. B., & Keizer, H. A. (2000). Exercise and Insulin Sensitivity: A Review. International Journal of Sports Medicine, 21(1), 1-12. Retrieved August 29, 2014.

10. Steigler, P. (2006). The Role of Diet and Exercise for the Maintenance of Fat-Free Mass and Resting Metabolic Rate during Weight Loss. Sports Medicine, 36(3), 239-262.

11. Thomas, J., & Kravitz, L. (2014). Exercise Benefits People with Osteoarthritis. IDEA Fitness Journal, 11(4), 16-19.

12. You, T., Arsenis, N., Disanzo, B., & LaMonte, M. (2013). Effects of Exercise Training on Chronic Inflammation in Obesity. Sports Medicine, 43(4), 243-256.

13. Thomas, J., & Kravitz, L. (2014). Exercise Benefits People with Osteoarthritis. IDEA Fitness Journal, 11(4), 16-19.

14. Ann Marie W. Petersen, Bente Klarlund; The anti-inflammatory effect of exercise Pedersen Journal of Applied Physiology Published 1 April 2005 Vol. 98 no. 4, 1154-1162 DOI:10.1152/japplphysiol.00164.2004.

15. M. Gleeson, N.C. Bishop, DJ Stensel - Nature Reviews, 2011 - nature.com

16. You, T., Arsenis, N., Disanzo, B., & LaMonte, M. (2013). Effects of Exercise Training on Chronic Inflammation in Obesity. Sports Medicine, 43(4), 243-256.

17. Hawley, J. A. (2004). Exercise as a therapeutic intervention for the prevention and treatment of insulin resistance. Diabetes/Metabolism Research and Reviews, 20(5), 383-393.

18. Myers, J. (2003). Exercise and Cardiovascular Health. Circulation, 107. Retrieved August 12, 2014, from http://circ.ahajournals.org/content/107/1/e2.short.

19. Bray, G. A. (2008). Good Calories, Bad Calories by Gary Taubes. Obesity Review 9(10), 251-263.

20. Clinic Staff. (2014, August 2). Metabolism and weight loss: How you burn calories. Mayo Clinic. Retrieved September 10, 2014.

21. Behm, D. G. (1995). Neuromuscular Implications and Applications of Resistance Training. The Journal of Strength and Conditioning Research, 9(4).

22. Hultman, E. (1995). Fuel Selection, Muscle Fibre. The Proceedings of the Nutrition Society, 1(54), 21-107.

23. Kraemer, W. J., & Gordon, S. (1991). Endogenous Anabolic Hormonal and Growth Factor Responses to Heavy Resistance Exercise in Males and Females. International Journal of Sports Medicine, 12(2), 228-235. Retrieved August 12, 2014.

24. Chalabaev, A., Emile, M., Corrion, K., Stephan, Y., Clément-Guillotin, C., Pradier, C., & d'Arripe-Longueville, F. (2013). Development and Validation of the Aging Stereotypes and Exercise Scale. Journal of Aging & Physical Activity, 21(3), 319-334.

25. Blumenthal, J. A., Babyak, M. A., Moore, K. A., Craighead, W. E., Herman, S., Khatri, P., et al. (1999). Effects of exercise training on older patients with major depression. Arch. Intern. Med. 159, 2349–2356.

26. Borg, G. (1990). Psychophysical scaling with applications in physical work and the perception of exertion. Scand. J. Work Environ. Health 16(Suppl. 1), 55–58.

27. Bouchard, C., and Rankinen, T. (2001). Individual differences in response to regular physical activity. Med. Sci. Sports Exerc. 33, S446–S451.

28. Burdette, J. H., Laurienti, P. J., Espeland, M. A., Morgan, A., Telesford, Q., Vechlekar, C. D., et al. (2010). Using network science to evaluate exercise-associated brain changes in older adults. Front. Aging Neurosci. 2:23.

29. Chapman, S. B., Aslan, S., Spence, J. S., Hart, J. J., Bartz, E. K., Didehbani, N., et al. (2013). Neural mechanisms of brain plasticity with complex cognitive training in healthy seniors. Cereb. Cortex. doi: 10.1093.

30. Chen, J. J., Rosas, H. D., and Salat, D. H. (2011). Age-associated reductions in cerebral blood flow are independent from regional atrophy. Neuroimage 55, 468–478.

31. Colcombe, S. J., Erickson, K. I., Scalf, P. E., Kim, J. S., Prakash, R., McAuley, E., et al. (2006). Aerobic exercise training increases brain volume in aging humans. J. Gerontol. A Biol. Sci. Med. Sci. 61, 1166–1170.

32. Colcombe, S. J., Kramer, A. F., Erickson, K. I., Scalf, P., McAuley, E., Cohen, N. J., et al. (2004). Cardiovascular fitness, cortical plasticity, and aging. Proc. Natl. Acad. Sci. U.S.A. 101, 3316–3321.

33. Conti, A. A., and Macchi, C. (2013). Protective effects of regular physical activity on human vascular system. Clin. Ter. 164, 293–294.

34. Dregan, A., and Gulliford, M. C. (2013). Leisure-time physical activity over the life course and cognitive functioning in late mid-adult years: a cohort-based investigation. Psychol. Med. 43, 2447–2458.

35. Erickson, K. I., Voss, M. W., Prakash, R. S., Basak, C., Szabo, A., Chaddock, L., et al. (2011). Exercise training increases size of hippocampus and improves memory. Proc. Natl. Acad. Sci. U.S.A. 108, 3017–3022.

36. Hillman, C. H., Erickson, K. I., and Kramer, A. F. (2008). Be smart, exercise your heart: exercise effects on brain and cognition. Nat. Rev. Neurosci. 9, 58–65

37. Horne, J. (2013). Exercise benefits for the aging brain depend on the accompanying cognitive load: insights from sleep electroencephalogram. Sleep Med. 14, 1208–1213.

38. Kadoglou, N. P., Fotiadis, G., Athanasiadou, Z., Vitta, I., Lampropoulos, S., and Vrabas, I. S. (2012). The effects of resistance training on ApoB/ApoA-I ratio, Lp(a) and inflammatory markers in patients with type 2 diabetes. Endocrine 42, 561–569.

39. Macintosh, B. J., Crane, D., and Rajab, A. S. (2012). Cerebral blood flow changes associated with a single aerobic exercise session. ISMRM Scientific Workshop Oral Session 4, 39.

40. Prakash, R. S., Snook, E. M., Motl, R. W., and Kramer, A. F. (2010). Aerobic fitness is associated with gray matter volume and white matter integrity in multiple sclerosis. Brain Res. 1341, 41–51.

41. Schaie, K. W., and Strother, C. R. (1968). A cross-sequential study of age changes in cognitive behavior. Psychol. Bull. 70, 671–680.

42. Shay, K. A., and Roth, D. L. (1992). Association between aerobic fitness and visuospatial performance in healthy older adults. Psychol. Aging 7, 15–24.

43. Shibata, S., and Levine, B. D. (2012). Effect of exercise training on biologic vascular age in healthy seniors. Am. J. Physiol. Heart Circ. Physiol. 302, H1340–H1346.

44. Steinhaus, L. A., Dustman, R. E., Ruhling, R. O., Emmerson, R. Y., Johnson, S. C., Shearer, D. E., et al. (1988). Cardio-respiratory fitness of young and older active and sedentary men. Br. J. Sports Med. 22, 163–166.

45. Tzourio-Mazoyer, N., Landeau, B., Voss, M. W., Prakash, R. S., Erickson, K. I., Basak, C., Chaddock, L., Kim, J. S., et al. (2010). Plasticity of brain networks in a randomized intervention trial of exercise training in older adults. Front. Aging Neurosci. 2:32.

CHAPTER TWO: Fat Is Skinny

1. Gunnars, K., "6 Graphs That Show Why The 'War' on Fat Was a Huge Mistake." Accessed January 7th, 2014.

2. Siri-Tarino, PW. et al., "Meta-analysis of prospective cohort studies evaluating the association of saturated fat with cardiovascular disease." Am J Clin Nutr January 2010 ajcn.27725.

3. Rong, Y. et al., "Egg consumption and risk of coronary heart disease and stroke: dose-response meta-analysis of prospective cohort studies." BMJ 2013; 346:e8539

4. Howard BV. et al., "Low-fat dietary pattern and weight change over 7 years: the Women's Health Initiative Dietary Modification Trial." JAMA. 2006 Jan 4; 295(1):39-49.

5. Stamler, J. et al., "Multiple Risk Factor Intervention Trial: Risk Factor Changes and Mortality Results." JAMA. 1982; 248(12):1465-1477.

6. Brehm BJ. et al., "A Randomized Trial Comparing a Very Low Carbohydrate Diet and a Calorie-Restricted Low Fat Diet on Body Weight and Cardiovascular Risk Factors in Healthy Women" J Clin Endocrinol Metab. 2003 Apr; 88(4):1617-23.

7. Lopez-Garcia, E., et al, "Consumption of Trans Fatty Acids Is Related to Plasma Biomarkers of Inflammation and Endothelial Dysfunction. J. Nutr. March 1, 2005 vol. 135 no. 3 562-566.

8. WHO technical report series 916. Diet, nutrition and the prevention of excess weight gain and obesity. Report of a joint WHO/FAO expert consultation. Geneva: WHO, 2003.

9. Swinburn BA, Caterson I, Seidell JC, James WP. Diet, nutrition and the prevention of excess weight gain and obesity. Public Health Nutr 2004; 7:123–46.

10. French SA, Story M, Jeffery RW. Environmental influences on eating and physical activity. Annu Rev Public Health 2001; 22:309–35.

11. Popitt SD, Prentice AM. Energy density and its role in the control of food intake: evidence from metabolic and community studies. Appetite 1996; 26:153–74.

12. Prentice AM, Jebb SA. Fast foods, energy density and obesity: a possible mechanistic link. Obes Rev 2003; 4:187–94.

13. Bowman SA, Gortmaker SL, Ebbeling CB, Pereira MA, Ludwig DS. Effects of fast-food consumption on energy intake and diet quality among children in a national household survey. Pediatrics 2004; 113:112–8.

14. Zizza C, Siega-Riz AM, Popkin BM. Significant increase in young adults' snacking between 1977–1978 and 1994–1996 represents a cause for concern! Prev Med 2001; 32:303–10.

15. Bray GA, Nielsen SJ, Popkin BM. Consumption of high-fructose corn syrup in beverages may play a role in the epidemic of obesity. Am J Clin Nutr2004; 79:537–43.

16. Berkey CS, Rockett HR, Field AE, Gillman MW, Colditz GA. Sugar-added beverages and adolescent weight change. Obes Res 2004; 12:778–88. Medline

17. Wiehe S, Lynch H, Park K. Sugar high: the marketing of soft drinks to America's schoolchildren. Arch Pediatr Adolesc Med 2004; 158:209–11.

18. Rolland-Cachera MF, Deheeger M, Akrout M, Bellisle F. Influence of macronutrients on adiposity development: a follow up study of nutrition and growth from 10 months to 8 years of age. Int J Obes Relat Metab Disord 1995; 19:573–8.

19. Brand-Miller JC, Holt SH, Pawlak DB, McMillan J. Glycemic index and obesity Am J Clin Nutr 2002; 76:281S–5S.

20. DiMeglio DP, Mattes RD. Liquid versus solid carbohydrate: effects on food intake and body weight. Int J Obes Relat Metab Disord 2000; 24:794–800.

21. Caraher M, Coveney J. Public health nutrition and food policy. Public Health Nutr 2004; 7:591–8.

22. Jacobson MF, Brownell KD. Small taxes on soft drinks and snack foods to promote health. Am J Public Health 2000; 90:854–7.

23. Fried EJ, Nestle M. The growing political movement against soft drinks in schools. JAMA 2002; 288:2181.

24. WHO report. Global strategy on diet, physical activity and health. World Health Organization. April 2004.

25. Cade J, Upmeier H, Calvert C, Greenwood D. Costs of a healthy diet: analysis from the UK Women's Cohort Study. Public Health Nutr 1999; 2:505–12.

26. Drewnowski A. Fat and sugar: an economic analysis. J Nutr 2003; 133:838S–40S.

27. Drewnowski A, Specter SE. Poverty and obesity: the role of energy density and energy costs. Am J Clin Nutr 2004; 79:6–16.

28. Drewnowski A. Energy intake and sensory properties of food. Am J Clin Nutr 1995; 62:1081S–5S.

29. Drewnowski A. Energy density, palatability, and satiety: implications for weight control. Nutr Rev 1998; 56:347–53.

30. Shepherd R. Resistance to changes in diet. Proc Nutr Soc 2002; 61:267–72.

31. Story M, Neumark-Sztainer D, French S. Individual and environmental influences on adolescent eating behaviors. J Am Diet Assoc 2002; 102(suppl 3):S40–S51.

32. Oh, sweet reason. The Economist vol 371, no 837, April 17–23, 2004.

33. Carpenter KJ. A short history of nutritional science: part 4 (1945–1985). J Nutr 2003; 133:3331–42.

34. Drewnowski A. The role of energy density. Lipids 2003; 38:109–15.

35. Gibson SA. Associations between energy density and macronutrient composition in the diets of pre-school children: sugars vs. starch. Int J Obes Relat Metab Disord 2000; 24:633–8.

36. Brunner EJ, Marmot MG, Nanchahal K, et al. Social inequality in coronary risk: central obesity and the metabolic syndrome. Evidence from the Whitehall II study. Diabetologia 1997; 40:1341–9.

37. Mokdad AH, Ford ES, Bowman BA, et al. Prevalence of obesity, diabetes, and obesity-related health risk factors, 2001. JAMA 2003; 289:76–79.

38. US Department of Health and Human Services. Healthy people 2010 report.

39. Yanovski S. Sugar and fat: cravings and aversions. J Nutr 2003; 1 33:835S–7S.

40. Levine AS, Kotz CM, Gosnell BA. Sugars and fats: the neurobiology of preference. J Nutr 2003; 133:831S–4S.

41. Blundell JE, MacDiarmid JI. Passive overconsumption. Fat intake and short-term energy balance. Ann NY Acad Sci 1997;827:392–407.

42. Rolls BJ, Castellanos VH, Halford JC. Volume of foods consumed affects satiety in men. Am J Clin Nutr 1998; 67:1170–7.

CHAPTER THREE: Exercise, Activity, and Fat Burning

1. Shaw K, Gennet H, O'Rourke P, Del Mar C. Exercise for Overweight or Obesity. John Wiley & Sons; 2006. The Cochrane Collaboration.

2. Wu T, Gao X, Chen M, Van Dam RM. Long-term effectiveness of diet-plus-exercise interventions vs. diet-only interventions for weight loss: a meta-analysis: obesity Management. Obesity Reviews. 2009; 10(3):313–3233. Tjønna AE, Stølen TO, Bye A, et al. Aerobic interval training reduces cardiovascular risk factors more than a multitreatment approach in overweight adolescents. Clinical Science. 2009; 116(4):317–326.

3. Babraj JA, Vollaard NBJ, Keast C, Guppy FM, Cottrell G, Timmons JA. Extremely short duration high intensity interval training substantially improves insulin action in young healthy males. BMC Endocrine Disorders. 2009; 9, article no. 3:1–8.

4. Trapp EG, Chisholm DJ, Freund J, Boutcher SH. The effects of high-intensity intermittent exercise training on fat loss and fasting insulin levels of young women. International Journal of Obesity. 2008; 32(4):684–691.

5. Wisloff U, Stoylen A, Loennechen JP, et al. Superior cardiovascular effect of aerobic interval training versus moderate continuous training in heart failure patients: a randomized study. Circulation. 2007; 115(24):3086–3094.

6. Harmer AR, Chisholm DJ, McKenna MJ, et al. Sprint training increases muscle oxidative metabolism during high-intensity exercise in patients with type 1 diabetes. Diabetes Care. 2008; 31(11):2097–2102.

7. Boudou P, Sobngwi E, Mauvais-Jarvis F, Vexiau P, Gautier J-F. Absence of exercise-induced variations in adiponectin levels despite decreased abdominal adiposity and improved insulin sensitivity in type 2 diabetic men. European Journal of Endocrinology. 2003; 149(5):421–424.

8. Coppoolse R, Schols AMWJ, Baarends EM, et al. Interval versus continuous training in patients with severe COPD: a randomized clinical trial. European Respiratory Journal. 1999; 14(2):258–263.

9. Rognmo Ø, Hetland E, Helgerud J, Hoff J, Slørdahl SA. High intensity aerobic interval exercise is superior to moderate intensity exercise for increasing aerobic capacity in patients with coronary artery disease. European Journal of Cardiovascular Prevention and Rehabilitation. 2004; 11(3):216–222.

10. Gibala MJ, McGee SL. Metabolic adaptations to short-term high-intensity interval training: a little pain for a lot of gain? Exercise and Sport Sciences Reviews. 2008; 36(2):58–63.

11. Trapp EG, Chisholm DJ, Boutcher SH. Metabolic response of trained and untrained women during high-intensity intermittent cycle exercise. American Journal of Physiology. 2007; 293(6):R2370–R2375.

12. Bracken RM, Linnane DM, Brooks S. Plasma catecholaine and neprinc responses to brief intermittent maximal intensity exercise. Amino Acids. 2009; 36:209–217.

13. Christmass MA, Dawson B, Arthur PG. Effect of work and recovery duration on skeletal muscle oxygenation and fuel use during sustained intermittent exercise. European Journal of Applied Physiology and Occupational Physiology. 1999;80(5):436–447.

14. Zouhal H, Jacob C, Delamarche P, Gratas-Delamarche A. Catecholamines and the effects of exercise, training and gender. Sports Medicine. 2008; 38(5):401–423.

15. Rebuffe-Scrive M, Andersson B, Olbe L, Bjorntorp P. Metabolism of adipose tissue in intraabdominal depots of nonobese men and women. Metabolism. 1989; 38(5):453–458.

16. Crampes F, Beauville M, Riviere D, Garrigues M. Effect of physical training in humans on the responses of isolated fat cells to epinephrine. Journal of Applied Physiology. 1986; 61(1):25–29.

17. Riviere D, Crampes F, Beauville M, Garrigues M. Lipolytic response of fat cells to catecholamines in sedentary and exercise-trained women. Journal of Applied Physiology. 1989; 66(1):330–335.

18. Nevill ME, Holmyard DJ, Hall GM, et al. Growth hormone responses to treadmill sprinting in sprint- and endurance-trained athletes. European Journal of Applied Physiology and Occupational Physiology. 1996; 72(5-6):460–467.

19. Vuorimaa T, Ahotupa M, Häkkinen K, Vasankari T. Different hormonal response to continuous and intermittent exercise in middle-distance and marathon runners. Scandinavian Journal of Medicine and Science in Sports. 2008; 18(5):565–572.

20. Hoffman JR, Falk B, Radom-Isaac S, et al. The effect of environmental temperature on testosterone and cortisol responses to high intensity, intermittent exercise in humans. European Journal of Applied Physiology and Occupational Physiology. 1997; 75(1):83–87.

21. Bussau VA, Ferreira LD, Jones TW, Fournier PA. The 10-s maximal sprint: a novel approach to counter an exercise-mediated fall in glycemia in individuals with type 1 diabetes. Diabetes Care. 2006; 29(3):601–606.

22. Gaitanos GC, Williams C, Boobis LH, Brooks S. Human muscle metabolism during intermittent maximal exercise. Journal of Applied Physiology. 1993; 75(2):712–719.

23. Buchheit M, Laursen PB, Ahmaidi S. Parasympathetic reactivation after repeated sprint exercise. American Journal of Physiology. 2007; 293(1):H133–H141.

24. Mourot L, Bouhaddi M, Tordi N, Rouillon J-D, Regnard J. Short- and long-term effects of a single bout of exercise on heart rate variability: comparison between constant and interval training exercises. European Journal of Applied Physiology. 2004; 92(4-5):508–517.

25. Burgomaster KA, Heigenhauser GJF, Gibala MJ. Effect of short-term sprint interval training on human skeletal muscle carbohydrate metabolism during exercise and time-trial performance. Journal of Applied Physiology. 2006; 100(6):2041–2047.

26. Tomlin DL, Wenger HA. The relationship between aerobic fitness and recovery from high intensity intermittent exercise. Sports Medicine. 2001; 31(1):1–11.

27. Almuzaini KS, Potteiger JA, Green SB. Effects of split exercise sessions on excess post exercise oxygen consumption and resting metabolic rate. Canadian Journal of Applied Physiology. 1998; 23(5):433–443.

28. Kaminsky LA, Padjen S, LaHam-Saeger J. Effects of split exercise sessions on excess postexercise oxygen consumption. British Journal of Sports Medicine. 1990; 24(2):95–98.

29. Laforgia J, Withers RT, Gore CJ. Effects of exercise intensity and duration on the excess post-exercise oxygen consumption. Journal of Sports Sciences. 2006; 24(12):1247–1264.

30. Burgomaster KA, Howarth KR, Phillips SM, et al. Similar metabolic adaptations during exercise after low volume sprint interval and traditional endurance training in humans. Journal of Physiology. 2008; 84(1):151–160.

31. Tremblay A, Simoneau J-A, Bouchard C. Impact of exercise intensity on body fatness and skeletal muscle metabolism. Metabolism. 1994; 43(7):814–818.

32. Helgerud J, Høydal K, Wang E, et al. Aerobic high-intensity intervals improve VO2max more than moderate training. Medicine and Science in Sports and Exercise. 2007; 39(4):665–671.

33. Mourier A, Gautier J-F, De Kerviler E, et al. Mobilization of visceral adipose tissue related to the improvement in insulin sensitivity in response to physical training in NIDDM: effects of branched-chain amino acid supplements. Diabetes Care. 1997; 20(3):385–391.

34. Perry CGR, Heigenhauser GJF, Bonen A, Spriet LL. High-intensity aerobic interval training increases fat and carbohydrate metabolic capacities in human skeletal muscle. Applied Physiology, Nutrition and Metabolism. 2008; 33(6):1112–1123.

35. Talanian JL, Galloway SDR, Heigenhauser GJF, Bonen A, Spriet LL. Two weeks of high-intensity aerobic interval training increases the capacity for fat oxidation during exercise in women. Journal of Applied Physiology. 2007; 102(4):1439–1447.

36. Tjønna AE, Lee SJ, Rognmo Ø, et al. Aerobic interval training versus continuous moderate exercise as a treatment for the metabolic syndrome: a pilot study. Circulation. 2008; 118(4):346–354. Warburton DER, McKenzie DC, Haykowsky MJ, et al. Effectiveness of high-intensity interval training for the rehabilitation of patients with coronary artery disease. American Journal of Cardiology. 2005; 95(9):1080–1084.

37. Whyte LJ, Gill JMR, Cathcart AJ. Effect of 2 weeks of sprint interval training on health-related outcomes in sedentary overweight/obese men. Metabolism Clinical and Experimental. 2010; 59(10):1421–1428.

38. Dunn SL. Effects of exercise and dietary intervention on metabolic syndrome markers of inactive premenopausal women. University of New South Wales; 2009.

39. Little JP, Safdar A, Cermak N, Tarnopolsky MA, Gibala MJ. Acute endurance exercise increases the nuclear abundance of PGC-1 alpha in trained human skeletal muscle. American Journal of Physiology. 2010; 298(4):R912–R917.

40. Gibala MJ, McGee SL, Garnham AP, Howlett KF, Snow RJ, Hargreaves M. Brief intense interval exercise activates AMPK and p38 MAPK signaling and increases the expression of PGC-1a in human skeletal muscle. Journal of Applied Physiology. 2009; 106(3):929–934.

41. Tabata I, Nishimura K, Kouzaki M, et al. Effects of moderate-intensity endurance and high-intensity intermittent training on anaerobic capacity and VO2max Medicine and Science in Sports and Exercise. 1996; 28(10):1327–1330.

42. Gibala M. Molecular responses to high-intensity interval exercise. Applied Physiology, Nutrition, and Metabolism. 2009; 34(3):428–432.

43. Macdougall JD, Hicks AL, Macdonald JR, Mckelvie RS, Green HJ, Smith KM. Muscle performance and enzymatic adaptations to sprint interval training. Journal of Applied Physiology. 1998; 84(6):2138–2142.

44. Teixeira PJ, Going SB, Houtkooper LB, et al. Pretreatment predictors of attrition and successful weight management in women. International Journal of Obesity. 2004; 28(9):1124–1133.

45. Burgomaster KA, Hughes SC, Heigenhauser GJF, Bradwell SN, Gibala MJ. Six sessions of sprint interval training increases muscle oxidative potential and cycle endurance capacity in humans. Journal of Applied Physiology. 2005; 98(6):1985–1990.

46. Bilski J, Teległów A, Zahradnik-Bilska J, Dembiński A, Warzecha Z. Effects of exercise on appetite and food intake regulation. Medicina Sportiva. 2009; 13(2):82–94.

47. Rivest S, Richard D. Involvement of corticotropin-releasing factor in the anorexia induced by exercise. Brain Research Bulletin. 1990; 25(1):169–172.

48. Clausen JP. Effect of physical training on cardiovascular adjustments to exercise in man. Physiological Reviews. 1977; 57(4):779–815.

49. Boutcher SH, Dunn SL. Factors that may impede the weight loss response to exercise-based interventions. Obesity Reviews. 2009; 10(6):671–680.

50. Gibala M., "Molecular responses to high-intensity interval exercise." Appl Physiol Nutr Metab. 2009 Jun; 34(3):428-32.

51. VO2max: what do we know, and what do we still need to know Levine, B.D. Institute for Exercise and Environmental Medicine, Presbyterian Hospital of Dallas, TX 75231. The Journal of Physiology, 2008 Jan 1; 586(1):25-34. Epub 2007 Nov 15.

52. Di Donato, Danielle; West, Daniel; Churchward-Venne, Tyler; Breen, Leigh; Baker, Steven; Phillips, Stuart (2014). "Influence of aerobic exercise intensity on myofibrillar and mitochondrial protein synthe-

sis in young men during early and late postexercise recovery". American Journal of Physiology - Endocrinology and Metabolism 306 (9): E1025–E1032. doi:10.1152/ajpendo.00487.2013.

53. Elmahgoub, S. S., Calders, P., Lambers, S., Stegen, S. M., Van Laethem, C., & Cambier, D. C. (2011). The effect of combined exercise training in adolescents who are overweight or obese with intellectual disability: The role of training frequency. Journal of Strength and Conditioning Research, 25(8), 1.

CHAPTER 8: Men, Women, and Weight Loss

1. Kraemer, W. J., & Gordon, S. (1991). Endogenous Anabolic Hormonal and Growth Factor Responses to Heavy Resistance Exercise in Males and Females. International Journal of Sports Medicine, 12(2), 228-235. Retrieved August 12, 2014.

2. American College of Sports Medicine. ACSM's Guidelines for Exercise Testing and Prescription 7th Edition. Philadelphia, PA: Lippincott Williams & Wilkins, 2006.

3. Brownell, K.D. The LEARN Program for Weight Management 10th Edition, Dallas, TX: American Health Publishing Company, 2004.

4. Costain, L. and Croker, H. Helping individuals to help themselves. Proc Nutr Soc 2005; 64:89-96.

5. Dennis, K.E. Weight management in women. Nurs Clin N Am 2004; 39:231-241.

6. Despres, J.P., Pouliot, M.C., and Moorjani, S. Loss of abdominal fat and metabolic response to exercise training in obese women. Am J Physiol 1991; 261:E151-167.

7. Fabricatore, A.N., and Wadden, T.A. Treatment of obesity. Clin Diabetes 2003; 21(2); 67-72.

8. Finkelstein, E.A., Fiebelkorn, I.C., and Wang, G. National medical spending attributable to overweight and obesity: How much, and who's paying? Health Affairs 2003: W3; 219–226.

9. Hu, F.B., Manson, J.E., Stampfer, M.J., et al. Diet, lifestyle, and the risk of type 2 diabetes mellitus in women. N Engl J Med 2001: 345(11); 790–797.

10. Johnson, C.A., Corrigan, S.A., Dubbert, P.M., and Gramling, S.E. Perceived barriers to exercise and weight control practices in community women. Women Health 1990: 16; 177-191.

11. King, A.C., Taylor, C.B., Haskell, W.L., and DeBusk, R.F. Identifying strategies for increasing employee physical activity levels: findings from the Stanford/Lockheed exercise survey. Health Ed Q 1990: 17; 269-285.

12. Klem, M.L., Wing, R.R., McGuire, M.T., Seagle, H.M., and Hill, J.O. A descriptive study of individuals successful at long-term maintenance of substantial weight loss. Am J Clin Nutr 1997: 66; 239-246.

13. National Center for Health Statistics. Health, United States, 2006. U.S. Department of Health and Human Services.Thompson, D., Brown, J.B, Nichols, G.A., Elmer, P.J., and Oster, G. Body mass index and future healthcare costs: a retrospective cohort study. Obes Res 2001: 9(3); 210-218.

14. Myers, J. (2003). Exercise and Cardiovascular Health. Circulation, 107. Retrieved August 12, 2014, from http://circ.ahajournals.org/content/107/1/e2.short#cited-by

15. Clinic Staff. (2014, August 2). Metabolism and weight loss: How you burn calories. Mayo Clinic. Retrieved September 10, 2014, from http://www.mayoclinic.org/healthy-living/weight-loss/in-depth/metabolism/art-20046508

16. Behm, D. G. (1995). Neuromuscular Implications and Applications of Resistance Training. The Journal of Strength and Conditioning Research, 9(4). Retrieved August 12, 2014, from http://journals.lww.com/nsca-jscr/Abstract/1995/11000/Neuromuscular.

17. Hultman, E. (1995). Fuel Selection, Muscle Fibre. The Proceedings of the Nutrition Society, 1(54), 21-107.

18. Enoka, R., & Stuart, D. (1985). The contribution of neuroscience to exercise studies. Federation Proceedings, 44(7), 2279-2285. Retrieved August 12, 2014.

19. Myers, J. (2003). Exercise and Cardiovascular Health. Circulation, 107. Retrieved August 12, 2014.

20. Bray, G. A. (2008). Good Calories, Bad Calories by Gary Taubes. Obesity Review, 9(10), 251-263.

21. Clinic Staff. (2014, August 2). Metabolism and weight loss: How you burn calories. Mayo Clinic. Retrieved September 10, 2014.

22. Behm, D. G. (1995). Neuromuscular Implications and Applications of Resistance Training. The Journal of Strength and Conditioning Research, 9(4). Retrieved August 12, 2014.

23. Hultman, E. (1995). Fuel Selection, Muscle Fibre. The Proceedings of the Nutrition Society, 1(54), 21-107.

24. Kraemer, W. J., & Gordon, S. (1991). Endogenous Anabolic Hormonal and Growth Factor Responses to Heavy Resistance Exercise in Males and Females. International Journal of Sports Medicine, 12(2), 228-235. Retrieved August 12, 2014.

25. Chalabaev, A., Emile, M., Corrion, K., Stephan, Y., Clément-Guillotin, C., Pradier, C., & d'Arripe-Longueville, F. (2013). Development and Val-

idation of the Aging Stereotypes and Exercise Scale. Journal of Aging & Physical Activity, 21(3), 319-334.

CHAPTER NINE: The Aging Athelete in All of Us

1. Agre JC, Pierce LE, Raab DM, McAdams M, Smith EL. Light resistance and stretching exercise in elderly women: effect upon strength. Arch Phys Med Rehabil. 1988 Apr; 69(4):273-276.

2. Akima H, Kano Y, Enomoto Y, et al. Muscle function in 164 men and women aged 20-84 yr. Med Sci Sports Exerc. 2001; 33:220-226.

3. Alnaqeeb MA, Goldspink G. Changes in fibre type, number and diameter in developing and ageing skeletal muscle. J Anat. 1987; 153:31-45.

4. Asmussen E, Fruensgaard K, Norgaard S. A follow-up longitudinal study of selected physiologic functions in former physical education students-after forty years. J Am Geriatr Soc. 1975 Oct; 23(10):442-450.

5. Bassey EJ, Fiatarone MA, O'Neill EF, et al. Leg extensor power and functional performance in very old men and women. Clin Sci (Lond) 1992; 82:321-327.

6. Belman MJ, Gaesser GA. Ventilatory muscle training in the elderly. J Appl Physiol (1985) 1988 Mar; 64(3):899-905.

7. Blaivas M, Carlson BM. Muscle fiber branching—difference between grafts in old and young rats. Mech Ageing Dev. 1991; 60:43-53.

8. Blumenthal, J. A., Babyak, M. A., Moore, K. A., Craighead, W. E., Herman, S., Khatri, P., et al. (1999). Effects of exercise training on older patients with major depression. Arch. Intern. Med. 159, 2349-2356

9. Brooks SV, Faulkner JA. Effects of aging on the structure and function of skeletal muscle. In: Roussos C, editor. The Thorax. New York: Marcel Dekker, Inc; 1995. pp. 295-312.

10. Brooks SV, Faulkner JA. Skeletal muscle weakness in old age: underlying mechanisms. Med Sci Sports Exerc. 1994; 26:432-439.

11. Brown MC, Holland RL, Hopkins WG. Motor nerve sprouting. Annu Rev Neurosci. 1981; 4:17-42.

12. Buchman, A. S., Boyle, P. A., Wilson, R. S., Bienias, J. L., and Bennett, D. A. (2007). Physical activity and motor decline in older persons. Muscle Nerve 35, 354-362.

13. Campbell MJ, McComas AJ, Petito F. Physiological changes in ageing muscles. J Neurol Neurosurg Psychiatry. 1973; 36:174-182.

14. Chen HI, Kuo CS. Relationship between respiratory muscle function and age, sex, and other factors. J Appl Physiol (1985) 1989 Feb; 66(2):943-948.

15. Chesky JA, LaFollette S, Travis M, Fortado C. Effect of physical training on myocardial enzyme activities in aging rats. J Appl Physiol Respir Environ Exerc Physiol. 1983 Oct; 55(4):1349–1353.

16. Coggan AR, Spina RJ, King DS, et al. Skeletal muscle adaptations to endurance training in 60- to 70-yr-old men and women. J Appl Physiol. 1992; 72:1780–1786.

17. Colcombe, S. J., Erickson, K. I., Scalf, P. E., Kim, J. S., Prakash, R., McAuley, E., et al. (2006). Aerobic exercise training increases brain volume in aging humans. J. Gerontol. A Biol. Sci. Med. Sci. 61, 1166–1170.

18. Conboy IM, Rando TA. Aging, stem cells and tissue regeneration: lessons from muscle. Cell Cycle. 2005; 4:407–410.

19. Doherty TJ, Brown WF. The estimated numbers and relative sizes of thenar motor units as selected by multiple point stimulation in young and older adults. Muscle Nerve. 1993; 16:355–366.

20. Faulkner JA, Brooks SV, Zerba E. Muscle atrophy and weakness with aging: contraction-induced injury as an underlying mechanism. J Gerontol A Biol Sci Med Sci. 1995; 50 Spec No:124–129.

21. Faulkner JA, Larkin LM, Claflin DR, et al. Age-related changes in the structure and function of skeletal muscles. Clin Exp Pharmacol Physiol. 2007; 34:1091–1096.

22. Faulkner JA. Terminology for contractions of muscles during shortening, while isometric, and during lengthening. J Appl Physiol. 2003; 95:455–459

23. Fried LP. Conference on the physiologic basis of frailty. Aging (Milano) 1992; 4:251–265.

24. Frontera WR, Hughes VA, Lutz KJ, et al. A cross-sectional study of muscle strength and mass in 45- to 78-yr-old men and women. J Appl Physiol. 1991; 71:644–650.

25. Frontera WR, Meredith CN, O'Reilly KP, et al. Strength conditioning in older men: skeletal muscle hypertrophy and improved function. J Appl Physiol. 1988; 64:1038–1044.

26. Frontera WR, Meredith CN, O'Reilly KP, Evans WJ. Strength training and determinants of VO2max in older men. J Appl Physiol (1985) 1990 Jan; 68(1):329–333.

27. Frontera WR, Meredith CN, O'Reilly KP, Knuttgen HG, Evans WJ. Strength conditioning in older men: skeletal muscle hypertrophy and improved function. J Appl Physiol (1985) 1988 Mar; 64(3):1038–1044.

28. Gollnick PD, Timson BF, Moore RL, et al. Muscular enlargement and number of fibers in skeletal muscles of rats. J Appl Physiol. 1981; 50:936–943.

29. Goodpaster BH, Park SW, Harris TB, et al. The loss of skeletal muscle strength, mass, and quality in older adults: the health, aging and body composition study. J Gerontol A Biol Sci Med Sci. 2006; 61:1059–1064.

30. Grimby G, Saltin B. The ageing muscle. Clin Physiol. 1983; 3:209–218.

31. Haddad F, Roy RR, Zhong H, et al. Atrophy responses to muscle inactivity. I. Cellular markers of protein deficits. J Appl Physiol. 2003; 95:781–790.

32. Hagberg JM, Graves JE, Limacher M, Woods DR, Leggett SH, Cononie C, Gruber JJ, Pollock ML. Cardiovascular responses of 70- to 79-yr-old men and women to exercise training. J Appl Physiol (1985) 1989.

33. Hagberg JM, Seals DR, Yerg JE, Gavin J, Gingerich R, Premachandra B, Holloszy JO. Metabolic responses to exercise in young and older athletes and sedentary men. J Appl Physiol (1985) 1988 Aug; 65(2):900–908.

34. Heath GW, Hagberg JM, Ehsani AA, et al. A physiological comparison of young and older endurance athletes. J Appl Physiol. 1981; 51:634–640.

35. Holloszy JO. Workshop on Sarcopenia: Muscle Atrophy in Old Age. J Gerontol. 1995; 50A:1–161.

36. Hooper AC. Length, diameter and number of ageing skeletal muscle fibres. Gerontology. 1981; 27:121–126.

37. Jones DA, Rutherford OM. Human muscle strength training: the effects of three different regimens and the nature of the resultant changes. J Physiol (Lond) 1987; 391:1–11.

38. Kadhiresan VA, Hassett CA, Faulkner JA. Properties of single motor units in medial gastrocnemius muscles of adult and old rats. J Physiol (Lond) 1996; 493(Pt 2):543–552.

39. Kanda K, Hashizume K, Nomoto E, et al. The effects of aging on physiological properties of fast and slow twitch motor units in the rat gastrocnemius. Neurosci Res. 1986; 3:242–246.

40. Kasch FW, Boyer JL, Van CS, et al. Cardiovascular changes with age and exercise. A 28-year longitudinal study. Scand J Med Sci Sports. 1995; 5:147–151.

41. Katz S, Branch LG, Branson MH, Papsidero JA, Beck JC, Greer DS. Active life expectancy. N Engl J Med. 1983 Nov 17; 309(20):1218–1224.

42. Klitgaard H, Brunet A, Maton B, Lamaziere C, Lesty C, Monod H. Morphological and biochemical changes in old rat muscles: effect of increased use. J Appl Physiol (1985) 1989 Oct; 67(4):1409–1417.

43. Klitgaard H, Marc R, Brunet A, Vandewalle H, Monod H. Contractile properties of old rat muscles: effect of increased use. J Appl Physiol (1985) 1989 Oct; 67(4):1401–1408.

44. Korhonen MT, Cristea A, Alen M, et al. Aging, muscle fiber type, and contractile function in sprint-trained athletes. J Appl Physiol. 2006; 101:906–917.

45. Lexell J, Taylor CC, Sjostrom M. What is the cause of the ageing atrophy? Total number, size and proportion of different fiber types studied in whole vastus lateralis muscle from 15- to 83-year-old men. J Neurol Sci. 1988; 84:275–294.

46. Lexell J. Human aging, muscle mass, and fiber type composition. J Gerontol. 1995; 50A:11–16.

47. MacDougall JD, Elder GC, Sale DG, et al. Effects of strength training and immobilization on human muscle fibres. Eur J Appl Physiol Occup Physiol. 1980; 43:25–34.

48. Marti B, Howald H. Long-term effects of physical training on aerobic capacity: controlled study of former elite athletes. J Appl Physiol. 1990; 69:1451–1459.

49. Marti B. Health benefits and risks in sports: the other side of the coin. Schweiz Rundsch Med Prax. 1989; 78:290–294.

50. Maud PJ, Pollock ML, Foster C, et al. Fifty years of training and competition in the marathon: Wally Hayward, age 70-a physiological profile. S Afr Med J. 1981; 59:153–157.

51. Maughan RJ, Watson JS, Weir J. Strength and cross-sectional area of human skeletal muscle. J Physiol (Lond) 1983; 338:37–49.

52. Maxwell LC, Faulkner JA, Hyatt GJ. Estimation of number of fibers in guinea pig skeletal muscles. J Appl Physiol. 1974; 37:259–264.

53. Mendias CL, Marcin JE, Calerdon DR, et al. Contractile properties of EDL and soleus muscles of myostatin-deficient mice. J Appl Physiol. 2006; 101:898–905.

54. Meredith CN, Frontera WR, Fisher EC, Hughes VA, Herland JC, Edwards J, Evans WJ. Peripheral effects of endurance training in young and old subjects. J Appl Physiol (1985) 1989 Jun; 66(6):2844–2849.

55. Mitchell PJ, Johnson SE, Hannon K. Insulin-like growth factor I stimulates myoblast expansion and myofiber development in the limb. Dev Dyn. 2002; 223:12–23.

56. Morey MC, Cowper PA, Feussner JR, DiPasquale RC, Crowley GM, Kitzman DW, Sullivan RJ., Jr Evaluation of a supervised exercise program in a geriatric population. J Am Geriatr Soc. 1989 Apr; 37(4):348–354.

57. Naso F, Carner E, Blankfort-Doyle W, Coughey K. Endurance training in the elderly nursing home patient. Arch Phys Med Rehabil. 1990 Mar; 71(3):241–243.

58. Paffenbarger RS, Jr, Hyde RT, Wing AL, et al. Physical activity, all-cause mortality, and longevity of college alumni. N Engl J Med. 1986; 314:605–613.

59. Paffenbarger RS, Jr, Hyde RT, Wing AL, Hsieh CC. Physical activity, all-cause mortality, and longevity of college alumni. N Engl J Med. 1986 Mar 6; 314(10):605–613.

60. Pearson SJ, Young A, Macaluso A, et al. Muscle function in elite master weightlifters. Med Sci Sports Exerc. 2002; 34:1199–1206.

61. Petrella JK, Kim JS, Cross JM, et al. Efficacy of myonuclear addition may explain differential myofiber growth among resistance-trained young and older men and women. Am J Physiol Endocrinol Metab. 2006; 291:E937–E946.

62. Pollock ML, Foster C, Knapp D, et al. Effect of age and training on aerobic capacity and body composition of master athletes. J Appl Physiol. 1987; 62:725–731.

63. Pollock ML, Mengelkoch LJ, Graves JE, et al. Twenty-year follow-up of aerobic power and body composition of older track athletes. J Appl Physiol. 1997;82:1508–1516.

64. Pollock ML, Miller HS, Jr, Wilmore J. Physiological characteristics of champion American track athletes 40 to 75 years of age. J Gerontol. 1974; 29: 645–649.

65. Posner JD, Gorman KM, Gitlin LN, Sands LP, Kleban M, Windsor L, Shaw C. Effects of exercise training in the elderly on the occurrence and time to onset of cardiovascular diagnoses. J Am Geriatr Soc. 1990 Mar; 38(3):205–210.

66. Robinson S, Dill DB, Robinson RD, et al. Physiological aging of champion runners. J Appl Physiol. 1976; 41: 46–51.

67. Robinson S, Dill DB, Robinson RD, Tzankoff SP, Wagner JA. Physiological aging of champion runners. J Appl Physiol. 1976 Jul; 41(1):46–51.

68. Robinson S, Dill DB, Tzankoff SP, Wagner JA, Robinson RD. Longitudinal studies of aging in 37 men. J Appl Physiol. 1975 Feb; 38(2):263–267.

69. Robinson S. Experimental studies of physical fitness in relation to age. Arbeitsphysiologie. 1938; 10:251–323.

70. Rogers MA, Hagberg JM, Martin WH, 3rd, Ehsani AA, Holloszy JO. Decline in VO2max with aging in master athletes and sedentary men. J Appl Physiol (1985) 1990 May; 68(5):2195–2199.

71. Shephard RJ. Management of exercise in the elderly. Can J Appl Sport Sci. 1984 Sep; 9(3):109–120.

72. Thompson RF, Crist DM, Marsh M, Rosenthal M. Effects of physical exercise for elderly patients with physical impairments. J Am Geriatr Soc. 1988 Feb; 36(2):130–135.

73. Tomonaga M. Histochemical and ultrastructural changes in senile human skeletal muscle. J Am Geriatr Soc. 1977 Mar; 25(3):125–131.

74. Toth MJ, Matthews DE, Tracy RP, et al. Age-related differences in skeletal muscle protein synthesis: relation to markers of immune activation. Am J Physiol Endocrinol Metab. 2005; 288:E883–E891.

75. Trappe S, Gallagher P, Harber M, et al. Single muscle fibre contractile properties in young and old men and women. J Physiol. 2003; 552:47–58.

76. Verdery RB. Failure to thrive in the elderly. Clin Geriatr Med. 1995; 11:653–659.

77. Verdijk LB, Koopman R, Schaart G, et al. Satellite cell content is specifically reduced in type II skeletal muscle fibers in the elderly. Am J Physiol Endocrinol Metab. 2007; 292:E151–E157.

78. Wilson GJ, Newton RU, Murphy AJ, et al. The optimal training load for the development of dynamic athletic performance. Med Sci Sports Exerc. 1993; 25: 1279–1286.

79. Young A, Stokes M, Crowe M. The size and strength of the quadriceps muscles of old and young men. Clin Physiol. 1985; 5: 145–154.

ABOUT THE AUTHOR

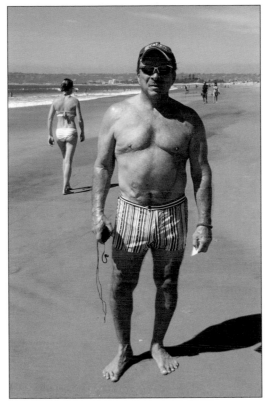

Dr. Ben at the beach in 2015

Dr. Vincent "Ben" Bocchicchio has worked professionally in the fields of fitness and health for nearly 40 years. An acknowledged leader in the field, he has built his success by combining science with effective body conditioning and technology to produce optimum health, fitness, rehabilitation, and weight loss for every body type. In the 1970s, Dr. Ben developed slow resistance training, a fitness technique that changed the way people exercise.

Dr. Ben grew up in Staten Island, New York, where he was an award-winning athlete in high school and college. His involvement in athletics inspired him to pursue a career in exercise science. He graduated in 1971 from Ithaca College with a bachelor's degree in physical education, health, and science. Dr. Ben went on to earn a master's degree in exercise sciences from Florida Atlantic University, a doctorate in exercise physiology from North American University, and a doctorate in health services, with a specialization in physical exercise, from Walden University. He also completed a postdoctoral program at Columbia University in body composition analysis and weight management.

In 1973 Dr. Ben founded a sports conditioning facility in Staten Island to condition professional and world-class athletes. Dr. Ben then applied the principles he developed for the athletic population, Slow MAximum Response Training or SMaRT™, to develop programs for weight reduction, cosmetic enhancement, general fitness, and health and rehabilitation for the general public. By 1978 Dr. Ben was lauded by the NY Press as "The Guru of Fitness."

He has served as an expert consultant to professional college teams and major sports conditioning programs, The US Olympic Committee, The National Football League, Major League Baseball, World Team Tennis, numerous major college athletic programs, and served as the training program developer for Total Gym®. In the early 1980s, Dr. Ben founded Cardio Management Systems and used resistance training as an integral part of Phase 2 Cardiac Rehabilitation. This was the first formally documented use of such exercise in the industry, and it is now commonplace protocol.

Following that experience, Dr. Ben became the exercise physiologist for Lehrman Back Centers in Miami Beach, Florida, a multi-phased, medical rehabilitation destination. He instituted his training protocol to become one of the leading consultants in the area of corporate fitness. His clients included Cardio Fitness Centers and The Vista Health Clubs for corporate fitness projects, the fitness club at the top of the World Trade Center, New York Health & Racquet Club, Gold's Gym, and World Gym International. Dr. Ben was also commissioned by Lutheran Medical Center and Staten Island University as well as a number of other teaching hospitals as the exercise physiologist for health, wellness, and weight-loss programs.

In addition, Dr. Ben became associated with OptiFast, the famous weight-loss program owned by Sandoz Medical that was made popular by Oprah Winfrey. He developed an adjunct exercise regimen called Opti Fit, using OptiFast patients as subjects in his second doctoral dissertation clinical trial. In that work, he established for the first time in scientific literature that long-term weight loss could not be accomplished without the incorporation of exercise. His paper, "The Development of Obesity and Fat Related Disorders," still stands as one of the only documents that accounts for the multi-dimensional nature of obesity and fat problems and addresses the proper application of exercise in every instance of origin.

Dr. Ben continues his research work in the fields of fitness, wellness, and health and has patented The FIRST exercise system program and trademarked his SMaRT-EX® system, which is also licensed and in use throughout the world.

The owner and operator of numerous health and fitness facilities throughout the nation, Dr. Ben currently maintains a private fitness and health practice in Phoenix, Arizona. His metabolic makeover program includes a proprietary exercise regimen, nutritional counseling, and EECP (Externally Enhanced Counter Pulsation). The results of these programs have been presented and scrutinized at meetings in the scientific community and have been clinically proven to be among the most effective available for body fat reduction, increased muscle tissue and metabolic rate levels, cardiovascular conditioning, and strength. All programs include sound, scientifically based, nutritional counseling to effect better health.

Dr. Ben has conducted and published studies in the fields of exercise and health and presented them to International Meetings of The American College of Sports Medicine and The American Physiological Society. He has authored more than two hundred articles, studies, and professional presentations on the subjects of health fitness and exercise and is cited in numerous books, articles, and studies as an expert. In 2009 Dr. Ben presented one study of clients who used his Metabolic Makeover techniques that demonstrated a reversal of the diabetic profile of Type II Diabetes in twelve weeks. He is currently working with Johns Hopkins Medical School as an investigator and consultant on two studies utilizing his slow resistance training concept for Juvenile Arthritic (JIA) patients and elderly patients with inflammatory disorders.

In his 60s, Dr. Ben continues to train regularly using his revolutionary SMaRT™ training system and maintains a high level of strength, significant muscle mass, and single digit body fat. He splits his time between Phoenix, Arizona, and Coronado, California.

SPECIAL OFFER!

Thanks for making the purchase of *15 Minutes to Fitness* by Dr. Ben Bocchicchio. Just by reading the book you have taken an important step to positively impacting your life.

Now Dr. Ben has created a way for you to continue your journey to a positive and healthy lifestyle. As a special incentive to all *15 Minutes to Fitness* readers, Dr. Ben has arranged with Total Gym® for you to save an additional **15%** off the price of a new Total Gym FIT model machine and any and all accessories of Total Gym products. Take advantage of this offer and save hundreds of dollars just for purchasing this book!

All you need to do to get your discount is
place your order at **totalgymdirect.com/drbentg**

Please act fast, as this offer will expire January 1, 2018.

• • •

Thank you, and a happy and healthy life to all!